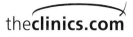
theclinics.com

NURSING CLINICS
OF NORTH AMERICA

Disaster Management and Response

GUEST EDITORS
Judith Stoner Halpern, MS, NP, APRN, BC and
Mary W. Chaffee, ScD (hon), MS, RN, CNAA, FAAN

September 2005 • Volume 40 • Number 3

SAUNDERS

An Imprint of Elsevier, Inc.
PHILADELPHIA   LONDON   TORONTO   MONTREAL   SYDNEY   TOKYO

W.B. SAUNDERS COMPANY
A Division of Elsevier Inc.

1600 John F. Kennedy Blvd., Suite 1800, Philadelphia, PA 19103-2899

http://www.theclinics.com

THE NURSING CLINICS OF NORTH AMERICA	Volume 40, Number 3
September 2005	ISSN 0029-6465
Editor: Maria Lorusso	ISBN 1-4160-2738-6

The ideas and opinions expressed in *The Nursing Clinics of North America* do not necessarily reflect those of the Publisher. The Publisher does not assume any responsibility for any injury and/or damage to persons or property arising out of or related to any use of the material contained in this periodical. The reader is advised to check the appropriate medical literature and the product information currently provided by the manufacturer of each drug to be administered to verify the dosage, the method and duration of administration, or contraindications. It is the responsibility of the treating physician or other health care professional, relying on independent experience and knowledge of the patient, to determine drug dosages and the best treatment for the patient. Mention of any product in this issue should not be construed as endorsement by the contributors, editors, or the Publisher of the product or manufacturers' claims.

The Nursing Clinics of North America (ISSN 0029-6465) is published quarterly by Elsevier Inc., Corporate and Editorial Offices: Elsevier Inc., 1600 John F. Kennedy Blvd., Suite 1800, Philadelphia, PA 19103-2899. Accounting and Circulation Offices: 6277 Sea Harbor Drive, Orlando, FL 32887-4800. Periodicals postage paid at Orlando, FL 32862, and additional mailing offices. Subscription price per year is, $100.00 (US individuals), $191.00 (US institutions), $165.00 (international individuals), $225.00 (international institutions), $138.00 (Canadian individuals), $225.00 (Canadian institutions), $55.00 (US students), and $83.00 (international students). To receive student/resident rate, orders must be accompanied by name of affiliated institution, date of term, and the signature of program/residency coordinator on institution letterhead. Orders will be billed at individual rate until proof of status is received. Foreign air speed delivery is included in all *Clinics* subscription prices. All prices are subject to change without notice. POSTMASTER: Send address changes to W.B. Saunders Company, Periodicals Fulfillment, Orlando, FL 32887-4800. **Customer Service: 1-800-654-2452 (US). From outside of the US, call 1-407-345-4000.**

Nursing Clinics of North America is covered in *EMBASE/Excerpta Medica, Index Medicus, Social Sciences Citation Index, Current Contents, ASCA, Cumulative Index to Nursing, RNdex Top 100*, and *Allied Health Literature and International Nursing Index (INI)*.

Printed in the United States of America.

NURSING CLINICS
OF NORTH AMERICA

Disaster Management and Response

GUEST EDITORS

JUDITH STONER HALPERN, MS, NP, APRN, BC, University of Michigan, School of Nursing, RN Studies, Ann Arbor, Michigan

MARY W. CHAFFEE, ScD (hon), MS, RN, CNAA, FAAN, Doctoral Student, PhD Program, Graduate School of Nursing, Uniformed Services University of the Health Sciences, Bethesda, Maryland

CONTRIBUTORS

GEORGIA BARTON, MA, RN, Adult Nurse Practitioner Student, University of Michigan School of Nursing, Ann Arbor, Michigan

RANDAL BEATON, PhD, EMT, Research Professor, Department of Psychosocial and Community Health, University of Washington School of Nursing, Seattle, Washington

SANDRA C. GARMON BIBB, DNSc, RN, Associate Professor, Graduate School of Nursing, Uniformed Services University of the Health Sciences, Bethesda, Maryland

CONNIE BOATRIGHT, MSN, RN, Bioterrorism and Emergency Management Program Manager, Indiana Primary Health Care Association; and National AMEDD Augmentation Detachment, US Army Reserve, Fort McPherson, Georgia

ELEANOR F. BOND, PhD, RN, FAAN, Professor, Department of Biobehavioral Nursing and Health Systems, University of Washington School of Nursing, Seattle, Washington

MARY W. CHAFFEE, ScD (hon), MS, RN, CNAA, FAAN, Doctoral Student, PhD Program, Graduate School of Nursing, Uniformed Services University of the Health Sciences, Bethesda, Maryland

FRANK L. COLE, PhD, RN, CEN, CS, FNP, FAAN, Professor of Nursing; Assistant Dean and Chair, Department of Acute and Continuing Care; and Director, Emergency Nurse Practitioner Education; The University of Texas Health Science Center at Houston, Houston, Texas

KEVIN DAVIES, RRC, MA, RN, PGCE, Principal Lecturer, School of Care Sciences, University of Glamorgan, Glyntaff, Pontypridd, South Wales, United Kingdom

PAT DEENY, RN, RNT, BSc (Hons) Nursing, Adv Dip Ed, Senior Lecturer in Nursing, University of Ulster, Magee Campus, Derry-Londonderry, Northern Ireland, United Kingdom

KAREN L. ELBERSON, PhD, RN, Associate Dean, Faculty Affairs; PhD Program Director; and Associate Professor, Graduate School of Nursing, Uniformed Services University of the Health Sciences, Bethesda, Maryland

RAY HIGGINSON, BN, RN, PGCE, Doctoral Student and Senior Lecturer, School of Care Sciences, University of Glamorgan, Glyntaff, Pontypridd, South Wales, United Kingdom

SUSAN McDANIEL HOHENHAUS, RN, MA, Pediatric Emergency Department, Duke University, Durham, North Carolina

BRIAN McFETRIDGE, RN, BSc (Hons) Nursing, Post Grad Cert Specialist Practice-Critical Care Nursing, Post Grad Dip Ed, Lecturer in Nursing, University of Ulster, Magee Campus, Derry-Londonderry, Northern Ireland, United Kingdom

K. JOANNE McGLOWN, RN, MHHA, CHE, PhD, University of Alabama at Birmingham, Birmingham, Alabama

ANN M. MITCHELL, PhD, RN, Assistant Professor of Nursing, University of Pittsburgh School of Nursing, Pittsburgh, Pennsylvania

ROSEMARIE ROWNEY, MPH, RN, Clinical Instructor, Schools of Nursing and Public Health; and Director of Training, Bioterrorism Preparedness Initiative, University of Michigan, Ann Arbor, Michigan

TERESA J. SAKRAIDA, DNSc, RN, Assistant Professor of Nursing, University of Pittsburgh School of Nursing, Pittsburgh, Pennsylvania

LYNN A. SLEPSKI, RN, MSN, CCNS, Doctoral Student, Graduate School of Nursing, Uniformed Services University of the Health Sciences, Bethesda, Maryland

JOAN M. STANLEY, PhD, RN, CRNP, FAAN, Director of Education Policy, American Association of Colleges of Nursing, Washington, District of Columbia; and Adult Primary Care Nurse Practitioner, Faculty Practice Office, University of Maryland Hospital, Baltimore, Maryland

PATRICIA HINTON WALKER, PhD, RN, FAAN, Dean and Professor, Graduate School of Nursing, Uniformed Services University of the Health Sciences, Bethesda, Maryland

ELIZABETH E. WEINER, PhD, RN, BC, FAAN, Senior Associate Dean for Educational Informatics; Professor of Nursing and Biomedical Informatics; and Associate Director, International Coalition for Mass Casualty Education, Vanderbilt University School of Nursing, Nashville, Tennessee

KIRSTYN K. ZALICE, MSN, CRNP, Clinical Assistant Professor of Nursing, Robert Morris University, School of Nursing and Allied Health, Moon Township, Pennsylvania

NURSING CLINICS
OF NORTH AMERICA

Disaster Management and Response

> Emergency preparedness is a concept frequently referred to within medical and psychological literature and in local, state, and federal documents, yet it is not well defined. There is no published theoretical or operational definition of the term, and no conceptual analysis of the phenomena of emergency preparedness exists within the literature. Because nursing is the single largest health professional resource for response, work toward further refinement of the concept of emergency preparedness has relevance for nursing practice. This article examines and attempts to clarify the concept of emergency preparedness, especially as it applies to nursing.

> Self, identity, and culture are important psychosocial concepts in the analysis of how individuals perceive self in social context, self across the lifespan, and self in relation to cultural context. Contemporary theories emphasize the importance of a holistic perspective and promote the idea of identity as opposed to self-concept. This article explores the application of these ideas to disasters to provide guidance for health care professionals on how disasters impact individuals, groups, and communities. Disasters have a major impact on social infrastructure and culture, and in turn result in a range of human responses. Placing identity and maintenance of cultural integrity at the heart of practice, health care professionals are encouraged to take a holistic perspective across all phases of the disaster. Individuals, groups, and communities exhibit a range of responses influenced by levels of vulnerability or resilience. Facilitating expression of feelings related to the disaster experience is an important focus for health care. Always working within the cultural context and being sensitive to the rituals related to remembering and mourning help preserve dignity and possibly facilitate creation of a new identity and a revised culture after a disaster.

Disaster Nursing Curriculum Development Based on Vulnerability Assessment in the Pacific Northwest

Eleanor F. Bond and Randal Beaton

Disasters caused by naturally occurring or deliberately caused infections, toxic chemical spills, radiologic releases, or other catastrophic events are likely to challenge the US health care system and pose special risks to vulnerable groups. Despite these threats in the environment, most US nursing programs lack disaster nursing content. This article describes disaster nursing competencies needed in Washington State based on standards, local geographic and population vulnerabilities, expert review, and surveys of nursing students and practicing nurses. Disaster nursing competencies included the following categories: (1) providing for patient care needs; (2) practicing safely; (3) preparing, implementing, and evaluating institutional and community protocols in preparation for a disaster; (4) reporting and communicating; and (5) accessing up-to-date information. Practicing nurses and student nurses indicated a strong need for disaster nursing content; the greatest perceived need was for content related to caring for injured or ill patients and practicing safely during a disaster.

Disaster Competency Development and Integration in Nursing Education

Joan M. Stanley

Nurses, because of their nursing education and perspective practicing in multiple roles and settings, are uniquely qualified for mass casualty preparedness and response. Educating the current 2.7 million registered nurses and all future nursing graduates is a daunting task. Nursing education must ensure that graduates are prepared with the necessary knowledge and skills for mass casualty incidents. Four key entities are essential for education's successful implementation of disaster preparedness: education and professional organizations, accreditation and regulatory bodies, schools of nursing, and continuing education providers. This article examines the role each of these key entities plays in the development of a nursing workforce prepared for mass casualty response. In addition, the International Nursing Coalition for Mass Casualty Education (INCMCE) registered nurse (RN) competencies for mass casualty incidents and guidelines for integrating these competencies into the nursing education curricula are presented.

A National Curriculum for Nurses in Emergency Preparedness and Response

Elizabeth E. Weiner

Preliminary and continuing education concerning emergency preparedness is needed for nurses. Although some nurses have had natural disaster training, most have not had training to respond to bioterrorism events. Several organizations are working to develop standards and curricula for such training. This article highlights these efforts.

Nurses need a comprehensive knowledge of doctrine, laws, regulations, programs, and processes that build the operational framework for health care preparedness. Key components of this knowledge base reside in the areas of: evolution of homeland security: laws and mandates affecting health care and compliance and regulatory issues for health care organizations. This article addresses primary components in both of these areas, after first assessing the status of nursing's involvement (in homeland security), as portrayed in the professional literature.

Public health services are vital to homeland security and defense, and nurses make up the majority of public health care workers. This article identifies issues in preparing for bioterrorism and describes the role of public health nurses in bioterrorism preparedness.

Advanced practice nurses (APNs) and nurse practitioners (NPs) have provided health care services during disasters; however, little appears in the literature about their role. APNs and NPs represent a significant portion of the nursing workforce. This article focuses on critical factors to consider when preparing and planning for the role of NPs.

Children have unique physiologic and developmental characteristics that need to be considered. Plans for pediatric care during mass casualty incidents (MCIs) need to be developed. This article highlights challenges in providing care to children after MCIs and provides considerations for providing pediatric care.

Disasters are tragic events that disrupt the normal functioning of a community and overwhelm personal and community resources. The people who experience or simply witness traumatic events can be affected emotionally and develop a range of physical and emotional responses, which in turn can produce psychological, social, and physiological dysfunction. The challenge for health care providers is to recognize the range of emotions and to be able to identify when professional help is indicated. This article provides an overview of the human stress response and describes sources of stress that follow disasters, acute stress disorder, post-traumatic stress disorder, and interventions and resources used to care for victims after disasters.

This article provides a perspective on the types of research questions that might be explored and strategies used in relation to disaster, terrorism, and mass casualty events. Research is addressed in the context of three areas of focus: issues related to the health care provider; issues affecting the patient, individual, family, and community; and issues related to the health care system.

The level of emergency preparedness in US hospitals is a concern in light of the steady threat of natural disasters, transportation and industrial accidents, and the possibility of terror attack resulting in mass casualties. The science of hospital emergency preparedness is in an early stage of development. For research to logically expand knowledge, an accurate assessment—or examination of the state of the science—is conducted to determine the current state of knowledge, gaps in knowledge, and opportunities for future research. Milsten reviewed the literature on hospital response to acute-onset disasters from 1977 to 1999. His review of 107 articles contains research studies, case studies, and lessons learned pieces largely published in the medical literature. Milsten's analysis provides a substantial starting point. This article examines Milsten's review, identifies articles that have been published that add to this knowledge base, and identifies additional phenomena of interest.

Although natural disasters are claiming fewer lives now than even as recently as 30 years ago, they remain responsible for many premature deaths, most in third-world countries. This article highlights the relationship of human factors that can be found with third-world disasters and reviews interventions that have been used to reduce illness, injuries and deaths.

NURSING CLINICS
OF NORTH AMERICA

Nurs Clin N Am 40 (2005) xiii–xv

NURSING CLINICS
OF NORTH AMERICA

ELSEVIER
SAUNDERS

PREFACE

Disaster Management and Response

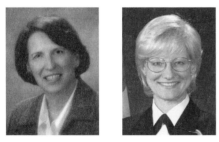

Judith Stoner Halpern, MS, NP, APRN, BC,
Mary W. Chaffee, ScD (hon), MS, RN, CNAA, FAAN

Guest Editors

D isasters are a continuous part of life on earth. Thousands were injured and killed in the Johnstown flood of 1889 and the Galveston hurricane of 1900. The Great New England Hurricane of 1938 caused over 500 deaths and at least 1700 injuries. The Kobe, Japan, earthquake of 1995 killed more than 500 people and injured nearly 27,000 others (how many urban health systems could handle that?). Thirty thousand people were injured in the Bam, Iran, earthquake in 2003. The death toll from the Asian tsunami is over 150,000; the total number of injured and homeless remains unclear.

The forces of nature are not the only cause of death and mass casualties. When the SS *Mont Blanc*, filled with munitions for the World War I exploded in Halifax, Nova Scotia, harbor in 1917, 9000 people were injured. The Hartford Circus Fire in 1944 sent about 480 burn victims in makeshift ambulances to Connecticut hospitals. The 1983 bombing of Harrod's Department store injured 94 people. Over 100,000 people were evacuated after the Chernobyl, Soviet Union, nuclear plant explosion in 1986, and more than 5 million people were exposed to radioactive fallout. When three Italian Air Force jets crashed at an air show in Ramstein, Germany, in 1988, 70 people were killed, and 450 people were injured. When United Airlines Flight 232 crash-landed at Sioux City, Iowa, in 1989, 112 people were killed, but 172 injured victims survived

0029-6465/05/$ – see front matter
doi:10.1016/j.cnur.2005.04.001

and needed emergency care. In 1996, the bombing of the Khobar Towers in Saudi Arabia, home to US military personnel and their families, resulted in 372 injuries. Hospitals in New York City treated nearly 800 injured victims between Sept. 11 and 13, 2001 after the World Trade Center bombing. Rescue workers made thousands of visits to health facilities during the rescue and recovery work in New York. Intentional food poisoning sent over 400 people to Nanjing, China, hospitals in 2002. When two trains crashed in Ryonchang, North Korea, in 2004, over 1300 people were injured.

Planning for the care of disaster victims is a challenge, because no one can predict where or when the next event will occur, only that there will be more. Disasters are by definition unpredictable, occur in different locations, are caused by different mechanisms, and, if they produce a large number of victims, they can place sudden and significant stresses on health care systems and health care workers.

Despite a long record of diverse disasters, some people are surprised by each new occurrence, possibly because of limited personal experience. If they have not lived through a hurricane, does that mean they never will? If a hospital has never been bombed in a community, does that mean local citizens can avoid preparation for such an unheard of event? If they have not seen a tornado, flood, or a volcanic eruption, does that mean they can remain blind to the possibility? The apparent disconnect between personal perception and reality has been identified as "disaster apathy" and can lead to an emergency preparedness posture that resembles an ostrich with its head in the sand.

Disaster preparedness requires resources: money, time, training, equipment, planning, exercise, and people. Many health care organizations find themselves squeezed in the center of dual pressures: preparedness versus profit. The right thing to do is not always the easy thing to do when finances are limited.

All health care providers have a role in disaster preparedness, especially nurses, who comprise the single largest workforce in the health sector. Nurses care for vulnerable populations and have a great opportunity to strengthen the level of emergency preparedness in their daily practice. No matter a nurse's specialty—clinician, educator, researcher, administrator, policy maker—each has the ability to provide direct input into how best to prepare for and provide disaster care. Disaster preparedness and response should be a part of every nurse's knowledge and skills.

This issue of *Nursing Clinics of North America* is designed to provide the reader with a variety of original articles that provide analysis and insight in many aspects of disaster health care. This issue is intended to assist in preparing nurses to respond effectively to disaster. The professional nurse needs to be a driving force in better preparing the nation, one patient, organization, and community at a time.

Judith Stoner Halpern, MS, NP, APRN, BC
University of Michigan, School of Nursing, RN Studies
400 North Ingalls
Ann Arbor, MI 48109-0482

E-mail address: jshalpern@charter.net

Mary W. Chaffee, ScD (hon), MS, RN, CNAA, FAAN
8601 Lime Kiln Court
Montgomery Village, MD 20886

E-mail address: mwchaffee@aol.com

Nurs Clin N Am 40 (2005) 419–430

NURSING CLINICS
OF NORTH AMERICA

Emergency Preparedness: Concept Development for Nursing Practice

Lynn A. Slepski, RN, MSN, CCNS*

Graduate School of Nursing, Uniformed Services University of the Health Sciences,
4301 Jones Bridge Road, Bethesda, MD 20814, USA

N ever before has the United States been so focused on improving its ability to respond to acts of terrorism. Ever since images appeared of commercial airliners driving into the World Trade Center and the Pentagon, Americans have felt vulnerable. US leaders, and leaders of other nations, have expressed great concern about levels of emergency preparedness, recognizing that large-scale events carry the potential for disastrous public health consequences. The threat of a large-scale incident is significant, and the United States remains dangerously unprepared. Recent terror events have killed thousands, placing the government's public health infrastructure under unprecedented scrutiny. These events highlight the need to connect the spheres of health care and emergency preparedness to each other and to the public. Emergency preparedness has become a national priority, and the federal government has responded by investing billions of dollars in preparedness.

Health care professionals have an obligation to treat as many victims with a chance of survival as possible during emergencies, but have they been lulled into complacency by the infrequency of events? Hospital personnel, those who face the challenge of organizing and implementing a plan to treat large numbers of casualties, have significant gaps in emergency preparedness knowledge and skills. Health care facilities are an essential component of the emergency response system, but they are poorly prepared for large-scale events. Finally, in most areas of the county, comprehensive community-wide emergency preparedness programs remain under development.

An intriguing situation has emerged. Weaknesses in the nation's preparedness, including many in the health sector, are being described and documented. Organizations are taking measures to improve preparedness. Colleges and universities are establishing new programs in various aspects of emergency preparedness and expanding current programs. But the target is not clear. What exactly is emergency preparedness?

* 102 Bristol Downs Drive, Gaithersburg, MD 20877, USA. *E-mail address*: lslepski@usuhs.mil

0029-6465/05/$ – see front matter   Published by Elsevier Inc.
doi:10.1016/j.cnur.2005.04.011   nursing.theclinics.com

THE CONCEPT OF EMERGENCY PREPAREDNESS

Emergency preparedness is addressed frequently in the health care and social sciences literature, and in local, state, and federal documents, but the concept is not defined well. The purpose of this concept analysis is to examine and clarify the concept of emergency preparedness, especially as it applies to nursing. Currently, no conceptual analysis of the phenomena of emergency preparedness exists. The concept will be reviewed in accordance with the Walker and Avant concept analysis technique [1].

LITERATURE REVIEW

The terrorist attacks in September 2001 and the subsequent anthrax attacks exposed weaknesses in the public health infrastructure and drew US policymakers' attention to the need for strengthened public health emergency preparedness at the local level [2]. As a result, several groups are examining the issues and implementing programs aimed at enhancing response capability [3].

The term emergency preparedness has been used as the basis for individual, local, state, and national preparedness plans aimed at enhancing readiness, increasing the ability to respond to large numbers of casualties by creating surge capacity, and improving the response to terrorism and other public health emergencies. The achievement of emergency preparedness takes place through a process that involves planning, training, and practicing skills through exercises, in addition to procuring equipment [4]. The federal government, in conjunction with state and local authorities, has taken unprecedented steps to enhance preparedness on multiple levels [5].

Little has been written about emergency preparedness. A search using PubMed, Cumulative Index for Nursing and Allied Health, and Psych INFO search engines and the term "emergency preparedness" resulted in no matches. Further searches using "disaster," "preparedness," "emergency," and similar related terms provided limited results, with most articles identified being related to natural and technological disasters.

Health care professionals and public health professionals are considered by many to be the first line of emergency defense [6–8]. The goal of this care is to deliver acceptable quality while saving as many lives as possible [9]. Little is known, however, about the level of health workforce preparedness nationwide [3,10]. The Gilmore Commission [3] found that many agencies and organizations implemented workforce preparedness activities without first conducting a needs assessment including baseline knowledge levels or learning styles of the audience or effective teaching methods. According to Vastag [11], physicians and nurses lack training; he states "physicians are not trained, paid or required to know about bioterrorism" [11]. Stanley [12] identified the 2.7 million nurses registered to practice in the United States as the single largest health professional resource for response and cites their expert assessment skills, critical thinking, decision-making and abilities to set priorities and collaborate as the greatest strengths they bring to managing emergencies.

Nurses are known to be team players and work effectively in the interdisciplinary teams needed in emergency situations [13].

Macintyre and colleagues [14] contend that many health-related emergency preparedness issues have not been addressed fully. Health care providers and facilities are vital collaborators in response to actual emergencies, yet they often are overlooked in the development of comprehensive community-wide emergency preparedness plans [14,15]. For example, Treat and colleagues [16] found that none of 30 hospitals examined were prepared to handle a biologic incident, and only 27% were prepared to handle a chemical incident. Approximately three fourths believed their sites were not prepared at all. Every hospital in their study reported a need for specific training but identified obstacles in achieving it.

Education and workforce training goals and strategies for emergency preparedness vary widely [2]. No standards are defined clearly, and guidelines for emergency preparedness do not exist [5,17]. Waeckerle [18] stated that there is no single source of authority or approved body of emergency preparedness content or curriculum, and as a result, there has been unfocused training and educational efforts. He noted that there is no program or policy office to integrate federal programs for emergency preparedness-related assistance and provide guidance to states and local communities. As Turnock [15] pointed out, the responsibility for defining what types and quantities of services are needed and what outcomes are desired and realizing them has been left to the states, raising the potential for inconsistency and lack of standardization of approaches from state to state. This may be because of the absence of an operational definition of emergency preparedness; without one, it is impossible to design the required education, training, and exercises to achieve it.

Wright [19] defines core competencies as the "knowledge, skills, abilities, and behaviors needed to carry out a job." In the absence of federal criteria, several groups independently have attempted to develop core competencies for emergency preparedness without attempting to coordinate the competencies across the many types of emergency responders. Health care roles already addressed include emergency medical technicians and physicians [20], hospital workers [21], and public health workers [21,22]. Groups addressing nursing core competencies include the American Red Cross [23], Association of Teachers of Preventive Medicine [24], and the International Nursing Coalition for Mass Casualty Education [25]. Unfortunately the vision and resulting core competency requirements are inconsistent across the groups.

Finally, emergency preparedness is big business. In total, the Department of Homeland Security (DHS), Department of Health and Human Services (DHHS), and Department of Justice provided $13.1 billion from FY'02 to FY'04 in grants to first responders and state and local governments to prevent, respond to, and recover from potential acts of terrorism and other potential disasters [26]. These funds were used to purchase equipment and provide training to help first responders save lives. However, no measures of effectiveness (MOEs), the quantifiable management tools that provide a qualitative and quantitative means for measuring effectiveness, outcomes, and performance, exist for emergency preparedness [15,27]. According to the Gilmore Commission [3], "there are not yet widely agreed upon metrics by which to assess levels of preparedness among the medical and public health workforces...there is not even a single definition of a "prepared workforce," because there is no consensus on what being prepared is." Without effective MOEs, it is impossible to demonstrate that these huge expenditures have been beneficial and have resulted in any improvements in preparedness levels.

DEFINITION OF EMERGENCY PREPAREDNESS

Although there has been many uses of the term emergency preparedness, there appears to be high degree of uncertainly as to what the term means. Several key documents using the term emergency preparedness were reviewed for this article. These included: the Federal Response Plan [28], Emergency Responder Guidelines [29], National Incident Management System [30], Interim National Response Plan [31], National Response Plan [32], National Incident Management System Integration Center [33], and Personal Emergency Preparedness [34]. Only one definition of emergency preparedness, which referred to municipalities and not personnel, was found. According to Perry and Lindell [4],

> "Emergency preparedness refers to the readiness of a political jurisdiction to react constructively to threats from the environment in a way that minimizes the negative consequences of impact for the health and safety of individuals and the integrity and functioning of physical structures and systems."

The concept emergency preparedness was not found in any of several dictionaries consulted or in Roget's Thesaurus. There is no published theoretical or operational definition of the term emergency preparedness on which to base the development of specific competencies. In conducting an analysis of the terms however, Merriam-Webster [35] defines emergency as: "(1) an unforeseen combination of circumstances or the resulting state that calls for immediate action; (2) urgent need for assistance or relief." Preparedness is defined [35] as "the quality or state of being prepared; esp: a state of adequate preparation in case of war." The Federal Emergency Management Agency [36] defines preparedness as "knowing the warning signs and what to do during an emergency" and "plans or preparations taken before an emergency occurs to save lives and to help response-and-rescue operations".

Homeland Security Presidential Directive (HSPD)-8 [37] states:

> The terms "major disaster" and "emergency" have the meanings given in section 102 of the Robert T. Stafford Disaster Relief and Emergency Assistance Act...The term "preparedness" refers to the existence of plans, procedures, policies, training, and equipment necessary at the Federal, State, and local level to maximize the ability to prevent, respond to, and recover from major events. The term "readiness" is used interchangeably with preparedness.

The Robert T. Stafford Disaster Relief and Emergency Assistance Act states:

"Emergency" means any occasion or instance for which, in the determination of the President, Federal assistance is needed to supplement State and local efforts and capabilities to save lives and to protect property and public health and safety, or to lessen or avert the threat of a catastrophe in any part of the United States [38].

Landesman [7] defines emergency as "any natural or man-made situation that results in severe injury, harm, or loss of humans or property" and preparedness as:

"All measures and policies taken before an event occurs that allow for prevention, mitigation, and readiness. Preparedness includes designing warning systems, planning for evacuation and relocation, storing food and water, building temporary shelter, devising management strategies, and holding disaster drills and exercises. Contingency planning is also included in preparedness as well as planning for postimpact response and recovery."

During a series of interviews, representatives from key organizational stakeholders were asked to define the term emergency preparedness. Organizations included: the American Red Cross; the Center for Health Policy, Columbia University School of Nursing; the Commissioned Corps Readiness Force, DHHS; the Emergency Management Institute, DHS; the Emergency Preparedness Evaluation and Specialty Branch of the Health Resources and Services Administration, DHHS; the International Nursing Coalition for Mass Casualty Education; and the National Disaster Medical System Training Program, DHS. All of these organizations used the term emergency preparedness without having or providing an operational definition of the term. Steven Sharro from the Emergency Management Institute emphasized:

It's one of those a-priori base terms that is expected to be commonly understood. I may be wrong, but I'm not aware of any FEMA doctrine that formally defines the term "emergency preparedness" (Steven Sharro, Emmitsburg, MD, personal communication, 2004).

Perhaps Turnock best sums up the lack of consensus of a definition of emergency preparedness in his comments [15]:

"Currently, states are not clear about what is meant by preparedness and how it can be measured and recognized. In this definitional vacuum, states are left to fend for themselves, resulting in uneven and inconsistent approaches from state to state and from locality to locality within states."

DEFINING ATTRIBUTES

Defining attributes are those characteristics of a concept that appear over and over again. They help to name the occurrence of a specific phenomenon as differentiated from similar or related ones [1].

Defining attributes are person-specific and role-specific. Nancy McKelvey, Chief Nurse of the American Red Cross, echoes this thought by describing both role-specific technical skills and personal attributes. She stated [8], "nurses need assessment skills to assess the individual, the group and the environment, and adaptability." She also identified that nurses need to be flexible, creative, and able to work in frequently changing environments with many different disciplines without the usual technology and support. Riba and Reches [39], as a result of focus groups with Israeli nurses, included as additional attributes of emergency preparedness: accountability; active, creative, and effective decision-making and problem-solving; assertiveness; autonomous action; dedication; the desire to do the right thing; effective communication; knowing where and how to access additional information and resources; open-mindedness; recognizing and acknowledging personal strengths and limitations; and the ability to function as a member of a team.

There are no defined national technical emergency preparedness standards for nurses. Several groups have attempted to define the technical skills required by nurses for emergency preparedness [23–25] by defining core competencies. No consensus on a required technical skills set has been reached.

ANTECEDENTS

Antecedents are the events or actions that must be in place or occur before a concept can transpire [1]. Chen and colleagues [40] examined family physicians' beliefs about preparedness and defined the antecedents of emergency preparedness as: (1) the awareness of the environment, (2) the perceived threat of an emergency, and (3) engagement in the identification of training needs. Other authors supported these views and also included planning for response and training and exercise as practice to cement new requisite skills [10,41–45]. For clinicians to take personal action to obtain and then update and reinforce training, they must see the benefit. They must believe that there is a personal risk to themselves and their community and new or additional skills needed that they must learn and practice to sustain their competence.

CONSEQUENCES

Consequences are those events or incidents that occur as a result of the occurrence of the concept. They are useful in determining neglected ideas, variables, or relationships that may yield new research directions [1]. Riba and Reches [40] cited as consequences of emergency preparedness: (1) personal satisfaction, (2) sense of control, (3) sense of achievement, (4) sense of pride, and (5) competent decision-making. Most importantly, their nurses identified specialized training as providing them the means to function in their role during the chaos of the disaster.

EMPIRICAL REFERENTS

Empirical referents are classes or categories of phenomena that measure the concept or determine its presence in the real world [1]. No metrics exist that measure overall emergency preparedness. Reineck and colleagues [46] developed the Army Nurse Readiness Instrument, which estimates the level of individual readiness perceived by Army nurses. Only one instrument exists that examines domestic preparedness training for first responders [47]. To a lesser degree, after action reviews and lessons learned could be considered a proxy for empirical referents if their recommendations were implemented. The influence of individuals and systems on core practices, both in capacity and performance, should be measurable. The instruments to measure and evaluate them have not been established. Therefore, development of standardized metrics and measurement tools is critical to empirical assessment of emergency preparedness.

RELATED CONCEPTS

Related concepts demonstrate similar ideas to the concept being studied, but differ when examined closely [1]. There are several concepts related to emergency preparedness that are used interchangeably but appear to have varied meanings. These include all-hazards preparedness [37], bioterrorism preparedness [5], citizen preparedness [48], community emergency preparedness [4], community preparedness [49], disaster preparedness [23], disaster response [23], family preparedness [49], hospital preparedness [16], individual preparedness [49], national biodefense preparedness [5], nurse preparedness [8], public preparedness [5], public health emergency preparedness [50], public health preparedness [2,51], and terrorism preparedness [52]. Also mentioned is the concept of emergency management as "the process of preparing for, mitigating, responding to and recovering from an emergency" [53] and surge capacity as "the ability to expand care capabilities in response to sudden or more prolonged demand [54]. Although each of the related concepts shares some attributes of emergency preparedness, some are threat-specific. Others involve only specific elements, such as planning or response, and do not encompass the entire breadth of the term emergency preparedness.

MODEL CASE

The following is a model case constructed to illustrate the concept of emergency preparedness. A model case is a real-life example of the concept that includes all of the defining attributes of emergency preparedness and no other attributes [1].

At the entrance to a shopping mall, a hospital nurse senses a strong vibration and watches as shelves and fixtures start to sway and items begin to fall to the floor. Realizing that an earthquake is taking place, she quickly exits the building and returns to her car in the parking lot. In the safety of her car, the nurse turns on her radio and hears a broadcast emergency alert over the local radio station announcing a 5.8 earthquake 100 miles from her location. Initial reports indicate the quake has resulted in many casualties. The broadcaster announces that the local hospital emergency plan has been implemented and that all staff are being asked to report for duty. The nurse returns to her home and initiates her family emergency plan. Her husband and children each perform their planned and exercised roles, turning off gas and water lines at the main valves. Then they move to the designated family area containing supplies, including a first aid kit, flashlights and spare batteries, bedding, bottled water, and nonperishable foods that require little or no cooking and no refrigeration. Using a battery-operated portable radio, her husband monitors the local emergency radio station. The children amuse themselves with games and coloring books put aside for this situation. Assured that her family is safe and taken care of, the nurse quickly consults a review sheet of her hospital's emergency plan and then drives to her place of employment. She arrives at the prescribed hospital entrance and presents her emergency response credential. She reports to the reception area and accepts her assignment in the triage area. As the first health care professional at the triage site, she quickly implements the triage portion of the hospital disaster plan. She assumes command of the triage area and evaluates and sorts casualties to the appropriate treatment site. When a senior staff member arrives, the nurse relinquishes command and assumes the role of staff person, assisting in the triage process. When the flow of casualties stops, the nurse returns to the reception area, to be told that there are no additional needs and she is released from duty. Upon arriving home, she recounts her personal satisfaction in performing well. She attributes her success to the ability to capitalize on experiences gained from previous training and exercises. She states that her experiences resulted in her ability to appropriately assume and function in her role in her family's as well as the hospital's emergency plans, allowing her to meet her organization's mission.

This scenario reflects that everyone knew what to do, that plans made earlier were put into action and worked. As a result, family members were safe, and medical and health services were available and provided. Fig. 1 illustrates the concept of emergency preparedness.

PROPOSED DEFINITION OF EMERGENCY PREPAREDNESS

Based on the preceding analysis, a clarified definition of emergency preparedness is proposed:

> Emergency preparedness is the comprehensive knowledge, skills, abilities, and actions needed to prepare for and respond to threatened, actual, or suspected chemical, biological, radiological, nuclear or explosive incidents, man-made incidents, natural disasters, or other related events.

RELEVANCE FOR NURSING

According to Walker and Avant [1], development of a concept analysis can be useful for:

- Defining ambiguous terms used in theory, practice, education, and research; providing operational definitions grounded in a theoretical basis
- Understanding the underlying attributes of a concept
- Assisting in the development of research instruments and outcome measures

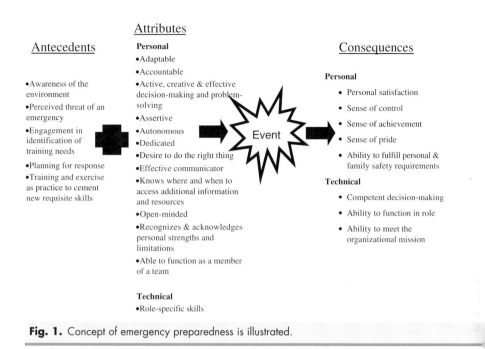

Fig. 1. Concept of emergency preparedness is illustrated.

Because nursing is the single largest health professional group, work toward further refinement of the concept of emergency preparedness has relevance for nursing practice and may assist in the development of research opportunities needed to understand this concept in its fullest dimension. Further studies are needed in a variety of settings and professional groups to assist in the development of nationally recognized and standardized core competencies.

SUMMARY

This concept analysis was undertaken to clarify the concept of emergency preparedness, enhance the application of theory to practice, and raise awareness of the responsibilities of the therapeutic role of health care providers in the emergency preparedness arena, especially nurses who engage in emergency preparedness activities. Although considerable progress has occurred since 2001, much remains to be done.

Consensus about the operational definition of emergency preparedness is fundamental to a comprehensive and effective national plan. Increased understanding of the concept will ensure that the range of preincident actions and processes are standardized and consistent with mutually agreed upon doctrine. More attention should be given to rigorous, scientific evaluation of the effectiveness of existing emergency preparedness training programs and the development of systems of metrics for measuring capacity and performance. These have significant implications for future research in this area. Although it is impossible to prevent future incidents, it is possible to set in place an emergency preparedness system that allows for activities to prepare for and respond to future emergencies, minimizing public health consequences.

References

[1] Walker LO, Avant KC. Strategies for theory construction. 3rd edition. Norwalk (CT): Appleton & Lange; 1995.

[2] US General Accounting Office. Bioterrorism: preparedness varied across state and local jurisdictions. Washington (DC): General Accounting Office; 2002.

[3] Gilmore Commission. Fourth annual report to the President and the Congress of the Advisory Panel to assess domestic response capabilities for terrorism involving weapons of mass destruction. Available at: http://www.rand.org/nsrd/terrpanel/terror4.pdf. Accessed December 19, 2003.

[4] Perry RW, Lindell MK. Preparedness for emergency response: guidelines for the emergency planning process. Disasters 2003;27(4):336–50.

[5] Council on Foreign Relations. Emergency responders: drastically underfunded, dangerously unprepared. Available at: http://www.cfr.org/pdf/Responders_TF.pdf. Accessed December 19, 2003.

[6] Bush GW. Biodefense for the 21st century. Speech. Washington (DC), February 11, 2004.

[7] Landesman LY, editor. Public health management of disasters: the practice guide. Washington (DC): The American Public Health Association; 2001.

[8] Veenema TG, editor. Disaster nursing and emergency preparedness for chemical, biological, and radiological terrorism and other hazards. New York: Springer; 2003.

[9] Levi L, Michaelson M, Admi H, et al. National strategy for mass casualty situation and its effects on the hospital. Prehospital Disaster Med 2002;17(1):12–6.

[10] Agency for Healthcare Research and Quality. Training of clinicians for public health events relevant to bioterrorism preparedness. Rockville (MD); 2002. Evidence Report/Technology Assessment, No. 51.

[11] Vastag B. Experts urge bioterrorism readiness. JAMA 2001;285(1):30–2.

[12] Stanley JM. Directions for nursing education. In: Veenema TG, editor. Disaster nursing and emergency preparedness for chemical, biological, and radiological terrorism and other hazards. New York: Springer; 2003. p. 461–71.

[13] Walker PH, Ricciardi R, Agazio JB. Directions for nursing research and development. In: Veenema TG, editor. Disaster nursing and emergency preparedness for chemical, biological, and radiological terrorism and other hazards. New York: Springer; 2003. p. 473–83.

[14] Macintyre AG, Christopher GW, Eitzen E, et al. Weapons of mass destruction events with contaminated casualties: effective planning for health care facilities. JAMA 2000; 283(2):242–9.

[15] Turnock BJ. Public health preparedness at a price: Illinois. New York: The Century Foundation; 2004.

[16] Treat KN, Williams JM, Furbee PM, et al. Hospital preparedness for weapons of mass destruction incidents: an initial assessment. Ann Emerg Med 2001;38(5):562–5.

[17] Everly GS. Thoughts on training guidelines in emergency mental health and crisis intervention. Int J Emerg Ment Health 2002;4(3):139–41.

[18] Waeckerle JA. Emergency departments: the Achilles heel of domestic preparedness. Presented at the Institute of Medicine's Future of Emergency Care Conference. Washington (DC), February 4, 2004.

[19] Wright D. The ultimate guide to competency assessment in healthcare. 2nd edition. Minneapolis (MN): Creative Healthcare Management; 1998.

[20] NBC Task Force. Final report: developing objectives, content and competencies for the training of emergency medical technicians, emergency physicians, and emergency nurses

to care for casualties resulting from nuclear, biological, or chemical (NBC) incidents. Washington (DC): US Government Printing Office; 2001.

[21] Columbia School of Nursing. Emergency preparedness competencies (annotated): public health professionals. New York: Center for Health Policy; 2001.

[22] Centers for Disease Control and Prevention. Bioterrorism & emergency readiness: competencies for all public health workers. Atlanta (GA): Centers for Disease Control and Prevention; 2002.

[23] American Red Cross. Introduction to disaster services. Washington (DC): American Red Cross; 2003.

[24] Association of Teachers of Preventive Medicine. Emergency response clinician competencies in initial assessment and management. New York: Center for Health Policy, Columbia University School of Nursing; 2003.

[25] International Nursing Coalition for Mass Casualty Education. Educational competencies for registered nurses responding to mass casualty incidents. Nashville (TN): International Nursing Coalition for Mass Casualty Education; 2003.

[26] Department of Homeland Security. Department of Homeland Security awards billions in grants to state and local governments. Available at: http://dhs.gov/dhspublic/display# theme=43&content=3416&print=true. Accessed March 30, 2004.

[27] Burkle FM. The concept of assisted management of large-scale disasters by horizontal organizations. Prehospital Disaster Med 2003;16(3):87–96.

[28] Federal Emergency Management Agency. The federal response plan. Washington (DC): US Government Printing Office; 1999.

[29] Department of Justice. Emergency responder guidelines. Washington (DC): Department of Justice; 2002.

[30] Department of Homeland Security. National incident management system. Washington (DC): Department of Homeland Security; 2003.

[31] Department of Homeland Security. Interim national response plan. Washington (DC): Department of Homeland Security; 2003.

[32] Department of Homeland Security. National response plan. Washington (DC): Department of Homeland Security; 2004.

[33] Department of Homeland Security. National incident management system integration center. Washington (DC): Department of Homeland Security; 2004.

[34] Department of Health and Human Services. Personal emergency preparedness. Atlanta (GA): Centers for Disease Control and Prevention; 2004.

[35] Merriam-Webster. Merriam-Webster collegiate dictionary. 10th edition. 2001. p. 918.

[36] Federal Emergency Management Agency. Emergency preparedness USA. Available at: http://training.fema.gov/EMIWeb/IS/is2lst.asp. Accessed December 19, 2003.

[37] White House. Homeland Security Presidential Directive/HSPD-8. Available at: http://www.whitehouse.gov/news/release/2003/12/print/20031217-6.html. Accessed December 19, 2003.

[38] Federal Emergency Management Agency. Robert T. Stafford Disaster Relief and Emergency Assistance Act [42 U.S.C. 5122, Section 102]. Available at: http://www.mwcog.org/security/security/otherplans/Stafford%20Act.pdf. Accessed December 19, 2003.

[39] Riba S, Reches H. When terror is routine: how Israeli nurses cope with multi-casualty terror. Online J Issues Nurs [serial online] 2002;7(3):manuscript 5. Available at: http://www.nursingworld.org/ojin/topic19_5.htm. Accessed June 22, 2004.

[40] Chen FM, Hickner J, Fink KS, et al. On the front lines: family physicians' preparedness for bioterrorism. J Fam Pract 2002;51(9):745–50.

[41] Agency for Healthcare Research and Quality. Training of hospital staff to respond to a mass casualty incident: summary. Rockville (MD); 2004. Evidence Report/Technology Assessment No. 95.

[42] Hilton C, Allison V. Disaster preparedness: an indictment for action by nursing educators. J Contin Educ Nurs 2004;35(2):59–65.

[43] Scharoun K, van Caulil K, Liberman A. Bioterrorism vs. health security—crafting a plan of preparedness. Health Care Manag 2002;21(1):74–92.

[44] Simpson D. Earthquake drills and simulations in community-based training and preparedness programmes. Disasters 2002;26(1):55–69.

[45] Winkenwerder W. Improving response to terror and global emerging infectious disease. Manag Care 2003;12(Suppl 11):2–6.

[46] Reineck C, Finstuen K, Connelly LM. Army nurse readiness instrument: Psychometric evaluation and field administration. Mil Med 2003;166(11):931–9.

[47] Beaton RD, Johnson C. Instrument development and evaluation of domestic preparedness training for first responders. Prehospital Disaster Med 2002;17(3):119–25.

[48] Department of Homeland Security. Department of Homeland Security launches citizen preparedness campaign. Available at: http://www.dhs.gov/dhspublic/display?theme=43&conentn=471&pring=true. Accessed May 15, 2004.

[49] Boy Scouts of America. Emergency preparedness: merit badge series. Irving (TX): Boy Scouts of America; 1995.

[50] Department of Health and Human Services. Strategic plan to combat bioterrorism and other public health threats and emergencies. Washington (DC): Department of Health and Human Services; 2003.

[51] McHugh M, Staiti AB, Felland LE. How prepared are Americans for public health emergencies? Twelve communities weigh in. Health Aff 2004;23(3):201–9.

[52] Department of Health and Human Services. A national public health strategy for terrorism preparedness and response 2003–2008. Atlanta (GA): Centers for Disease Control and Prevention; 2004.

[53] Federal Emergency Management Agency. Emergency management guide for business & industry. Washington (DC): Ogilvy, Adams & Rinehart; 2003.

[54] Joint Commission on the Accreditation Healthcare Organizations. Health care at the crossroads. Available at: http://www.jcaho.org/about+us/public+policy+initiatives/emergency+preparedness.pdf. Accessed June 22, 2004.

Nurs Clin N Am 40 (2005) 431–440

NURSING CLINICS
OF NORTH AMERICA

The Impact of Disaster on Culture, Self, and Identity: Increased Awareness by Health Care Professionals is Needed

Pat Deeny, RN, RNT, BSc (Hons) Nursing, Adv Dip Ed*,
Brian McFetridge, RN, BSc (Hons) Nursing,
Post Grad Cert Specialist Practice-Critical Care Nursing,
Post Grad Dip Ed

University of Ulster, Magee Campus, Northland Road, Derry-Londonderry,
Northern Ireland BT48 7HL, UK

Gist and Lubin [1] published the authoritative text on the psychosocial aspects of disaster in 1989. At that time, it was recognized that a community affected by a disaster is a community in transition. Experiencing a disaster means that a community may not be able to provide the individual with the necessary resources to deal with such extraordinary events [1]. Despite no direct reference to the importance of self, identity, and culture, there is recognition that a disaster impacts on the psychosocial functioning of individuals, groups, and communities. At times of great stress, the interrelatedness of individual, group, and community becomes more apparent.

Health care professionals must consider psychosocial impact when working with disaster survivors. Although it is important to focus on the life-preserving interventions in the acute phase, it would be short-sighted to ignore the psychosocial aspects of disasters and the impact they may have on the recovery and postrecovery phases. To achieve a holistic approach to health care, it is important to be aware of such issues, including the predisaster phase. Ignoring this, especially in the acute phase, undermines the idea that the total person is the focus of care.

Application of theories relating to self, identity, and culture reflects the idea that disasters impact at individual, group, and community levels. There is a paucity of empirical evidence that relates directly to these processes; however, it is possible to infer that health care professionals need to be aware of these fundamental concepts. This article explores the application of these ideas to health care practice in disasters and offers ideas for future developments. The

*Corresponding author. E-mail address: pg.deeny@ulster.ac.uk (P. Deeny).

0029-6465/05/$ – see front matter
doi:10.1016/j.cnur.2005.04.012

resilience of individuals and local communities to cope with extraordinary events must be appreciated. Within the philosophy of community empowerment, it must be recognized that individuals need to respond within their own cultural context. Health care professionals must have a flexible approach to helping at the scene of a disaster. They must work within existing community organizations and aim to enhance the response within these groups.

THE NATURE OF DISASTERS

A disaster is a calamitous event of slow or rapid onset that results in large-scale physical destruction of property, social infrastructure, and human life. It results in the existing resources and coping mechanisms of individuals, groups, communities, and societies being overwhelmed. The impact of the disaster may be determined strongly by the nature of the physical event, such as the loss of life and destruction of property. It is important to recognize, however, that the underlying factors such as lack of preparedness and poor infrastructure can make an equal contribution to the overall impact of the disaster [2–8]. Quarantelli, in the classic definition, outlines the importance of the imbalance in the demand–capability ratio [8]. It is this imbalance between the ability of the individual, group, or community to cope with the event that is central to understanding the concept of disaster. Disaster is multi-dimensional; it has all of the dynamic of any social issue, but superimposed on it is the degree of social disruption and the need to find an answer and meaning as to why the disaster occurred. The latter means that disaster affects culture and requires the mechanisms associated with culture to facilitate recovery.

During the last decade of the 20th century, an average of 75,250 people per year around the world lost their lives because of natural or human-initiated disasters. During the same period, 210 million people per year were affected by disasters [9]. Natural and human-initiated disasters always have been among the greatest risks to existence of the human race [10]. Since the events of Sept. 11, 2001, and the increasing threat of terrorist-related disasters, world awareness of disaster preparedness and response is probably at an all-time high. It is important, therefore, that health care professionals attend to this and become familiar with the psychosocial processes associated with disaster and the immediate life-saving requirements. Such awareness not only contributes to practice in the aftermath but also helps to enhance the capacity of groups and communities in disaster preparedness.

HOLISTIC AND TRANSCULTURAL PERSPECTIVES IN HEALTH CARE

In the immediate, and sometimes long-term, healthcare management tends to focus on dealing with physical needs. In the acute phase of a disaster, food, shelter, safe water, sanitation, and health services have to be delivered as soon as possible to save lives. It is possible that this may result in little attention being paid to discovering the specific needs of the community [11]. Health care professionals cannot afford to merely focus on the physical components of care without due consideration for the holistic needs of individuals and communities. Although this reductionist approach is vital in order to save lives, an approach with a transcultural and holistic philosophy should be used to support individual and cultural response to disaster.

In transcultural nursing theory, it is proposed that the value and belief components of cultures influence decision-making and actions within the culture. It is recognized that individuals are culturally unique, with cultural individuality being developed through life experiences, role modeling, and traits being passed on from past generations [12]. Such an approach is reflected in the international codes and standards that guide disaster management [5,13]. It is the essence of humanitarianism as described by the International Federation of Red Cross and Red Crescent Societies [5]. It also is recognized that humanitarianism often is presented as being about neutrality and impartiality. Disaster planning and management often involves intervention by national armies. Whatever the source of the intervention or the political beliefs of the group delivering the help, the same holistic approach is required. Health care from any source that does not display cultural sensitivity and appreciation of religious and traditional beliefs within groups will be met with resistance [11,12] and most likely will be ineffective.

THEORETICAL PERSPECTIVES ON SELF, IDENTITY, AND CULTURE

Self, identity, and culture are intertwined in how individuals feel about themselves and how they feel about living in a particular social context. The natural or human-initiated disaster has potential to seriously disrupt the life and social networks of individuals, groups, and communities. It is reasonable, therefore, to suggest that a disaster may result in changes related to self, identity, and culture. A presentation of the concepts will help to clarify this.

Since the introduction of the self concept and the consciousness of self in psychology [14], the study of how individuals perceive themselves in relation to others within a group or society remains an important focus in any discipline that places people at the center of activity or research. The literature on self, identity, and culture spans all of 20th century psychology and sociology. It includes the writings of the most eminent theorists in the field: Cooley (looking glass self) [15], Freud (ego psychology) [16], Mead (symbolic interaction role identity) [17], Erikson (developmental identity theory) [18], Kelly (personal construct theory) [19], Festinger (cognitive dissonance) [20], Marcia (identity and psychosocial development) [21], and Weinreich and Saunderson (identity structure analysis) [22]. This article provides only a brief outline of the concepts from these theorists, and practitioners will be made aware of recent and essential texts in the field.

The starting point for understanding of self, identity, and culture is the literature on the self and the self-concept. This provides evidence that people (either as individuals or as members of a group/culture/society) perceive self in a unique and complex way. The perception of self is a judgment on the part of the individual. It is a judgment that involves judging self in relation to others in a group, culture, or society. Moreover this perception of self is not limited to an evaluation of self in the social context. It includes the psychological processes associated with evaluation of self in relation to significant others, self across the life-span, self in relation to particular values and beliefs, and self in relation to a particular kinship and/or linage [23–26]. It is the introduction of these societal and cultural dimensions to the evaluation of self that has resulted in the term identity almost replacing the idea of a self-concept. Identity is much more holistic, as it is conceptualized as a broad biopsychosocial self-definition [26]. In this sense, it is much more applicable to disciplines such as health care professions that emphasize the holistic and transcultural approach.

Culture is used to describe the beliefs, ritual practices, art forms, ceremonies, and informal practices such as language, gossip, stories, and rituals of daily life [26]. It is a nebulous term that has been used broadly to describe almost all social processes. Culture can be seen as a behavioral response, which has been developed and influenced by social, religious, and intellectual manifestations [27]. Broad definitions of culture, however, make it difficult to analyze. Cote and Levine describe culture in a more focused way. Culture is comprised of the symbolic vehicles that facilitate the sharing of thoughts and behavior within a community. They go to propose that culture does not shape the identity of individuals absolutely but provides them with the resources to construct identity. Therefore, any change in social structure that results in disturbance in beliefs, ritual practices, art forms, and ceremonies will result in mitigation of the methods available for cultural expression and eventually the identity of individuals. This places culture at the center of the identity processes in coping with disasters [28].

EVALUATION OF THE EFFECT OF DISASTER ON SELF, IDENTITY, AND CULTURE

The examination of self, identity and culture in disasters is more implicit than explicit in the literature. Although there is a plethora of literature associated with psychosocial aspects of disaster, very little of it specifically relates to self, identity, and culture. This is surprising when the centrality of these ideas to psychological well-being is considered. Perhaps this could be rationalized by the view that these concepts have been developed at a theoretical level and have yet to be established as an empirical base for practice. The lack of available research on the topic results in an evaluation of the impact of disaster on self, identity, and culture being difficult.

For this reason, the literature pertaining to health care in disasters was scanned for themes that directly or tentatively relate to self, identity, and culture. Themes such as resilience and vulnerability, feelings associated with trauma, and remembrance and mourning emerge as being important. These themes merely act as a framework for discussion and a starting point for further debate and research. Each theme is discussed with the purpose of determining the impact of the disaster experience on self, identity, and culture and identifying points of importance for future practice.

Resilience and vulnerability

Individuals and communities have a natural ability to respond in a constructive manner to calamitous and traumatic events. This positive response in the face of adversity can be described as resilience. Balanced against this and on the opposite end of the continuum is the idea that individuals and communities have latent vulnerabilities. When considering individual or community response to disaster, this resilience–vulnerability continuum can be a valuable conceptual framework.

The concept of resilience describes how individuals or communities have the ability to respond and adapt in a positive manner to negative life experiences. Resilience is a dynamic process that occurs when normal activities are disrupted [29]. For resilience to be effective, there must be an ability to draw upon existing resources, knowledge and skills, while also being able to live and work in a challenging environment [30]. Being resilient does not suggest that individuals and cultures are not injured or damaged; rather, it explains how they adapt and recover [31]. Jacelon's examination of the concept of resilience indicated that individuals become resilient in two stages. The acute stage of the adversity requires immediate adaptation. The second stage is how the individual responds to the adversity over a longer period of time. These stages are crucial considerations in the health care professional's response in disasters. Certain personal characteristics, such high level of intelligence, problem-solving abilities, strong sense of self, positive outlook, and independence, may influence an individual's ability to be resilient positively [29].

In the disaster situation, health care professionals must be able to identify the prerequisites to resilience that exist within the community. Health care professionals must understand the area and culture and its previous experience of disasters. Once these are identified, the community and culture can be empowered to cope with the impact of the present disaster. Kendra and Wachtendorf emphasize that resilient communities can assist the responders to become resilient in their disaster management efforts. The resilient community will have important local knowledge and skills that may be valuable to the health care professional in helping to cope with the situation [32].

Vulnerability, on the other hand, describes the factors that may impair individual or community response. From the perspective of the health care professional, determining the vulnerabilities is equally if not more important than resilience. The degree of vulnerability may be the underpinning justification for intervention; hence it is important to have a clear idea where the vulnerabilities of a community lie. Such vulnerabilities range from the risk of a disaster occurring in the first place to the inability of the community to respond appropriately. Disasters in the developing world are a good illustration of the resilience–vulnerability continuum.

Most disasters occur in developing countries where there is lack of infrastructure and resources, endemic disease, conflicts, wars, and poverty [9]. This increases vulnerability and therefore requires intervention and support from richer countries. In relation to resilience, communities in developing countries may be good at coping simply because of their experiences of disasters. It is unwise to assume anything until proper consultation with the community and/or those who have knowledge of the local situation is made. At a fundamental level, health care professionals must strive to establish how individuals and communities can mitigate vulnerability with resilience. It is not easy to identify individual and community traits of resilience and vulnerability [30]. As is the case with most groups or cultures, it takes a long time before an outsider fully understands the attributes of the culture. This points to the need for preparedness when possible to invest necessary effort and resources, while also working alongside communities and cultural groups.

Feelings associated with trauma

Disasters often are associated with horrific and traumatic experiences. Whether such experiences are the result of the individual brush with death, witness to the death of others, torture, pain, or rape, the common denominator is some form of traumatic memory. Etched in the memory of the individual, the experience has potential to cause stress on an almost constant basis. Living with such memories of trauma can arrest development of the individual [33]. Not all individuals who experience trauma caused by a disaster have negative feelings, however. Only fifty percent will experience significant symptoms with which they will need assistance; 25% will go on to develop post-traumatic stress disorder (PTSD), and up to one third will develop chronic symptoms such as PTSD, anxiety, and depression [34]. These are generalizations. Figures will vary according to the scale of the disaster and resilience/vulnerability of the affected groups. An example of the psychological response of a community to disaster was following the 1994 Northridge earthquake [35]. Graves identified marked differences in the scope of emotional response depending on distance from the disaster. Communities closer to the higher-impact areas reported higher levels of psychological after effects (78%), whereas those further away had a lower percentage (54%) [35]. Surveys are valuable for providing quick impressions of disaster impact but do not inform thinking about the meaning of the disaster for the community.

Although it is accepted that exposure to disasters is likely to be extremely distressing, most people will cope quite well [36]. Health care professionals, however, should be alert to the underlying possibility of individuals developing stress reactions. In particular, they should be aware of the necessity to identify those at risk of developing a chronic stress reaction. Austin explains that lack of social support, the presence of pre-existing trauma, and the presence of pre-existing psychiatric problems all predict the development of chronic stress reactions [37]. As a traumatic event, the disaster experience impacts who people are, their identity, and how they view themselves within groups and community. Failure to recognize and deal with hurts and trauma can only result in poor mental health and impaired community functioning.

Remembrance and mourning

Disasters normally are associated with great loss, be it close family, friends, neighbors, the home, or sometimes a whole way of life. Remembrance and mourning are foremost in the initial stages after a disaster. Herman emphasizes the importance of remembrance and mourning, describing it as the second stage of recovery, once a safe environment and control have been re-established [33]. This is an invaluable framework for those health care professionals who are involved in direct therapeutic interventions with individuals or groups impacted by the disaster. It helps the therapist realize that there is an order to the process, and that patience and time are required to facilitate movement toward recovery. Evidence from Northern Ireland points to the assumption that individuals and communities get over the emotional impact. Approximately 50% of those impacted by the troubles in Northern Ireland still had symptoms of emotional distress, such sleep disturbance and health difficulties, over 20 years after the event. This study also highlights the difficulty in quantifying the number of individuals affected directly or indirectly by the traumatic events [38]. Whole families and communities are impacted by events. It is not limited to those directly involved.

In the disaster situation, not all health care professionals will possess bereavement counseling skills. Because existing counseling services may be overwhelmed, informal counseling may be provided by existing groups, individuals in the community, or family members. Help channeled through existing organizations is often more effective [7]. Health care professionals must identify existing formal support networks and provide victims with relevant referrals. Health care providers should focus on providing information and education to communities on the importance of telling their story or reconstructing the story. This reconstruction of the story [33] is not restricted to the immediate period after the disaster, but can extend for years. This is particularly important at remembrance events or in cases where there is a reoccurrence of a similar disaster. The Madrid bombings on March 11, 2004, likely have brought back painful memories for those affected by the Sept. 11, 2001, attacks in New York and Washington.

The stories of the Great Irish Famine, a disaster that resulted in the death of 4 million people in the mid-19th century still prevail in folklore in Ireland [39]. In their account of the aftermath of the Bhopal Disaster, Lapierre and Moro describe how the slum dwellers of Orya Shanty burn an effigy of the chairman of Union Carbide at the anniversary [40]. As part of the recovery process for the hundred-day massacre in Rwanda in 1994, it is commonplace for communities to hold an annual event that involves bone collecting. This involves bringing bones to the site of the atrocity. Each year different communities host the event and remember those who died. This event acts as a memorial and an opportunity for those who feel their family members may have been forgotten [41]. These are merely four examples of the many disasters that are now an integral part of the culture and history of the societies initially impacted. Stories of disasters exist for many years and are a necessary part of the overall identity of surviving individuals and communities.

At a more pragmatic level, someone has to deal with the dead and monitor the mortality levels. The International Federation of Red Cross and Red Crescent Societies in the 1997 World Disasters Report describe this role as the graveyard watch [5]. This role describes the importance of monitoring the level of deaths in the disaster zone and noting the uptake of burial shrouds and coffins if they exist. Alongside the practicalities of monitoring data relating to mortality figures, there is also a need for facilitating the normal rituals associated with death, burial, or cremation. In some disasters, quarantine restrictions and criminal investigation prevent release of the body to the family, which adds to the difficulties encountered by the family, community, and health care professionals. Although the latter normally is beyond the control of health care professionals in the field, an appreciation of the impact of this on the local culture is important. Mechanisms for keeping families updated on the living and dead will be required. Moreover, it is important to appreciate that the families that have been impacted by the disaster directly will need to participate in the funerals of others from the community. This can be demanding but a necessary feature of community recovery [42]. In Western cultures and agricultural communities, the death or quarantine of family pets and farm animals also can be stressful.

SUMMARY

As natural and human-initiated disasters continue to be a threat to individuals and communities, health care professionals have a responsibility to develop and improve preparedness and response to these events. Revisiting the definitions of disaster emphasizes that the disaster should not be examined primarily as physical, but also as a social and psychological phenomenon. The concepts of self, identity, and culture are important social and psychological phenomena, which are likely to be affected by the disaster experience. How the individual perceives self in social context and across a life span emerge as being important aspects of human existence. It is reasonable to suggest that human identity with all its dimensions (past, present, and future perspectives on self) and the inter-relatedness with culture would be disturbed by the disaster experience. Evidence is scanty, however, and until such time that researchers use ideas from identity theory as a conceptual framework, the position will remain the same.

Examining such concepts generates ideas that inform thinking on how best to approach the planning and management of health care in a disaster. Placing the person at the center of practice means that health care professionals must take account of the totality of the disaster experience. Individuals in a disaster situation remain entitled to the highest standard of care, albeit mitigated by lack of resources and disruption of infrastructure. The highest standard of care in the disaster situation as recognized by the sphere guidelines [13] emphasizes the importance of appreciating the local culture. As disasters often result in seeking or providing assistance from outside, it is imperative that such assistance does not add to the burden of the community. It is not the role of health care professionals to disturb the coping mechanisms that already exist but to enhance them. The importance of working closely with local communities, both in preparing for disaster and in disaster recovery, is emphasized. Intervention without due care and attention to the importance of identity and culture is inappropriate and contrary to humanitarian principles. Consulting with communities on their perceptions of resilience and vulnerability in relation to health care delivery at all phases of the disaster is valuable. There must be recognition that expressions of feelings that result from traumatic experiences are important. Such expression must be facilitated within the context of the local culture, and the needs of all groups must be addressed. Remembering and mourning can last for many years and may become established in a new identity and revised culture for individuals and communities after the disaster.

References
[1] Gist R, Lubin B. Psychosocial aspects of disaster. New York: John Wiley and Sons; 1989.
[2] World Health Organisation Regional Office for Europe. Humanitarian relief operations. EUR/RC43/15. Geneva (Switzerland): World Health Organisation; 1993.
[3] World Health Organisation. Emergency and humanitarian relief operation WHA46.6 agenda item 18.2. Geneva (Switzerland): World Health Organisation; 1993.
[4] Davies K, Deeny P, Raikkonnen M. A transcultural ethos underpinning curriculum development: a master's programme in disaster relief nursing. J Transcult Nurs 2003; 14(4):349–57.
[5] International Federation of Red Cross and Red Crescent Societies. World disasters report 1997; Geneva (Switzerland): IFRC; 1997.
[6] Drabek TE, McEntire DA. Emergent phenomena and the sociology of disaster: lessens, trends and opportunities from the research literature. Disaster Prevention and Management 2003;12(2):97–112.
[7] Eränen L, Leibkind K. Coping with disaster: the helping behaviour of communities and individuals. In: Wilson J, Rapheal B, editors. International handbook of traumatic stress syndromes. London: Plenum; 1993. p. 957–64.
[8] Quarantelli EL, editor. What is disaster? New York: Routledge; 1998.
[9] International Federation of Red Cross and Red Crescent Societies. World disasters report 2001: focus on recovery. Geneva (Switzerland): IFRC; 2001.
[10] Deeny P, Davies K, Gillespie M. International disaster nursing. In: Veenema TG, editor. Disaster preparedness and bioterrorism. New York: Springer; 2003. p. 484–95.
[11] Médecins Sans Frontières. Refugee health: an approach to emergency situations. London: MacMillan Education Limited; 1997.
[12] Leininger M, McFarland MR. Transcultural nursing: concepts, theories, research, and practice. 3rd edition. New York: McGrath-Hill; 2002.
[13] The Sphere Project. Humanitarian charter and minimum standards in disaster response. Geneva (Switzerland): The Sphere Project; 2004.
[14] James W. Principles of psychology. Cleveland (OH): World Publishing; 1892. Baumeister RF, editor. The self in social psychology. Philadelphia: Psychology Press; 1999. p. 69–77 [reprint].
[15] Cooley CH. human nature and the social order. New York: Scribner's; 1902.

[16] Freud S. The ego and the id. New York: Norton; 1923.

[17] Mead G, Mind H. Self and society. Chicago: University of Chicago Press; 1934.

[18] Erikison EH. Identity and the life cycle; selected papers. New York: International Universities Press; 1959.

[19] Kelly GA. The psychology of personal constructs. New York: Norton; 1955.

[20] Festinger L. A theory of cognitive dissonance. Stanford (CA): Stanford University Press; 1957.

[21] Marcia JE. Identity and psychosocial development in adulthood. Identity 2002;2(1):7–28.

[22] Weinreich P, Saunderson W, editors. Analysing identity: cross-cultural, societal and clinical contexts. New York: Routledge; 2003.

[23] Baumeister RF, editor. The self in social psychology. Philadelphia: Psychology Press; 1999.

[24] Billingham R, Hockey J, Strawbridge S. Exploring self and society. London: Macmillan Press; 1998.

[25] Breakwell G. Coping with threatened identities. London: Methuen & Company; 1986.

[26] Weinreich P. Identity structure analysis. In: Weinreich P, Saunderson W, editors. Analysing identity: cross-cultural, societal and clinical contexts. New York: Routledge; 2003. p. 7–76.

[27] Giger JN, Davidhizar RE. Transcultural nursing: assessment and intervention. St Louis (MO): Mosby; 1999.

[28] Cote JE, Levine GC. Identity formation, agency and culture; a social psychological synthesis. London: Lawrence Erlbaum Associates; 2002.

[29] Jacelon CS. The trait and process of resilience. J Adv Nurs 1997;25:123–9.

[30] Paton D, Johnston D. Disasters and communities: vulnerability, resilience and preparedness. Disaster Prevention and Management 2001;10(4):270–7.

[31] Kaniasty K, Norris FH. The experience of disaster: individuals and communities sharing trauma. In: Gist R, Lubin B, editors. Response to disaster; psychosocial, community and ecological approaches. Philadelphia: Taylor and Francis; 1999. p. 25–62.

[32] Kendra JM, Wachtendorf T. Elements of resilience after the World Trade Centre disaster: reconstituting New York City's emergency operation. Disasters 2003;27(1):37–53.

[33] Herman J. Trauma and recovery; the aftermath of violence-from domestic abuse to political terror. New York: Basic Books; 1997.

[34] Hodgkinson PE, Stewart M. Coping with catastrophe: a handbook of postdisaster psychosocial aftercare. London: Routledge; 1998.

[35] Graves JS. Emotional aftermath of a major earthquake: lessons for business. AAOHN Journal 1995;43(2):95–100.

[36] World Health Organisation. Mental health of populations exposed to biological and chemical weapons. Geneva (Switzerland): World Health Organisation; 2004.

[37] Austin LS. Responding to disaster: a guide for mental health professionals. Washington (DC): American Psychiatric Press Limited; 1992.

[38] Fay MT, Morrissey M, Smyth M, et al. The Cost of the Troubles Study: report on the Northern Ireland survey. The experience and impact of the troubles. Derry-Londonderry (UK): INCORE; 1999.

[39] Póirtéir C, editor. The great Irish famine. Dublin (Ireland): Mercer Press; 1995.

[40] Lapierre D, Moro J. Five past midnight in Bhopal. London: Scribner; 2003.

[41] Galete J. Postgenocide trauma counseling in Rwanda. Presented at the Program for Trocaire Seminar on Trauma Counselling. Belfast (Ireland), March 12, 2004.

[42] Englund H. Death, trauma and ritual: Mozambican refugees in Malawi. Soc Sci Med 1998;46(9):1165–74.

Nurs Clin N Am 40 (2005) 441–451

NURSING CLINICS
OF NORTH AMERICA

Disaster Nursing Curriculum Development Based on Vulnerability Assessment in the Pacific Northwest

Eleanor F. Bond, PhD, RN, FAAN*, Randal Beaton, PhD, EMT

University of Washington School of Nursing, 1959 Northeast Pacific Street, Box 357266, Seattle, WA 98195, USA

It seems probable that new infectious agents like sudden acute respiratory syndrome (SARS) will continue to emerge. Infections may be spread because of worldwide movement of people, or caused by unsanitary food preparation and distribution practices like the Pacific Northwest *Escherichia coli* 0157:H7 outbreaks, or from a deliberate attack like the East Coast anthrax cases of 2001. Toxic chemicals could poison a region's air, water, or food. Large numbers of casualties could result from a nuclear disaster. Natural disasters such as earthquakes, tsunamis, and floods have the potential to overwhelm community resources, including health care resources.

To respond effectively in all of these possible situations, nurses require adequate preparation. During a disaster, nurses are likely to function at the initiation of patient encounters. Nurses commonly provide leadership in development of institutional and community health care protocols. Nurses require knowledge and essential skills to work effectively during emergencies and disasters. However, this content is not included in nursing curricula. Recognizing the need for new learning opportunities, a project was undertaken to design curricular elements for Washington State nurses and nursing students. The purpose of this project was to formulate and validate competencies needed by nurses practicing in the Pacific Northwest region of the United States and to survey the interests of nursing students and practicing nurses related to their perceived need for disaster nursing content. This information would form a foundation for development of nursing-specific disaster curriculum. An important part of planning is the process of identifying

This project/was supported in part by funds from the Bureau of Health Professions (BHPr), Health Resources Services Administration (HRSA), Department of Health and Human Services (DHHS), under a grant (Bioterrorism Curriculum Development Program, number 1-T01-HP-00148 for $804,234). The information or content and conclusions are those of the authors and should not be construed as the official position or policy of, nor should be any endorsements be inferred by the BHPr, DHHS, or the US government.

*Corresponding author. *E-mail address:* rebond@u.washington.edu (E.F. Bond).

regional risks in a vulnerability analysis to determine what types of hazards the region's nurses are most likely to encounter.

DEFINING DISASTER

Disaster has been defined as an extraordinary event, either naturally occurring or contrived, that acutely challenges a system to deliver a rapid response and exceeding that system's usual response capacity [1]. A disaster is likely to disrupt essential services, including health care, sanitation, transportation, and law enforcement. Water and air quality also may be adversely affected.

VULNERABILITY ASSESSMENT OF THE PACIFIC NORTHWEST

To design curricular elements related to disaster nursing in Washington State, regional vulnerabilities were reviewed, and potentially vulnerable groups were identified. The Puget Sound area, densely populated and industrialized, is particularly vulnerable to disaster. Puget Sound industries include commercial and military aviation, biotechnology, and computer technology; each poses unique risks for accident or sabotage. The Boeing Company has 80,000 employees in Washington State. Boeing is one of the world's largest manufacturers of commercial and military aircraft and is one of the nation's largest National Aeronautics and Space Administration (NASA) contractors. Boeing fighter/attack products include fighter jets such as the Hornet, Super Hornet, F-15 Eagle, and F-18 Raptor, and rotorcraft including the Chinook, Apache, and Osprey. Toxic chemicals commonly used in commercial aeronautical manufacturing include cyanide and chlorine [2]. These have been identified as potential chemical weapons of opportunity [3]. Several major computer software companies are headquartered in the Puget Sound area also. Because of the iconic nature of the companies and the critical dependence of the business sector on their products, these corporations are considered potential targets for terrorist attacks.

Eco-terrorists are active in the Pacific Northwest. The Environmental Liberation Front (ELF), classified as domestic terrorists by the Federal Bureau of Investigation (FBI), is suspected in the destruction by arson of the University of Washington Center for Urban Horticulture building. The event did not impact public health, but it gives credence to the notion that this sector could instigate public health catastrophes. In January 2002, ELF released its 2001 annual report, in which it claimed responsibility for burning the Center for Urban Horticulture and for 137 other attacks/illegal acts including several other fires in Washington State.

The Puget Sound's vulnerability is enhanced, because it is a port of entry for vessels from the Pacific Rim and Canada and an import/export shipping hub for grain and manufactured goods. In November 2001, a traveler with suspected smallpox arrived at Seattle-Tacoma International Airport. Although the patient did not have smallpox, the incident demonstrated the need for systematic public health preparedness. In December 1999, a customs agent in Port Angeles, Washington, detected an Al Qaeda terrorist attempting to enter the United States from Canada. The terrorist arrived aboard an international ferry driving a carload of explosives. The event caused Seattle authorities to publicly acknowledge the region's vulnerability and to cancel public millennium celebrations. The defendant was later convicted in a Los Angeles court of plotting to bomb Los Angeles Airport [4].

A number of US military reservations are in the Puget Sound area. These include Fort Lewis (9th Infantry Division headquarters), Naval Air Station Whidbey Island, Submarine Base Bangor, Naval Station Bremerton, Naval Station Everett, McCord Air Force Base, and Fairchild Air Force Base. These bases have been active in recent Southwest Asia military responses, thus possibly subject to reprisal.

Approximately 150 miles east of Seattle and Tacoma, the aging Hanford Nuclear Facility poses the risk of environmental release because of accident or sabotage. The Hanford reservation is home to a commercial nuclear power plant and stores large amounts of radioactive nuclear waste.

There are five active or potentially active volcanoes in Washington State. Mount Saint Helens erupted in 1980, devastating more than 150 square miles of forest and recreation area, resulting in nearly 60 deaths. Mount Rainier is considered a dangerous volcano because of the large population living around its lowland drainages. Four urban centers, Seattle, Tacoma, and Olympia, Washington, and Portland, Oregon, are within 100 miles of Mount Rainier.

Early in 2001, the Puget Sound area experienced a major earthquake of magnitude 6.8 on Richter scale, and the area remains at risk for earthquake. Subsequent to this earthquake, a series of earthquakes in the Spokane surprised citizens and geologists, and altered risk estimates for earthquakes in the Pacific Northwest. Western Washington has numerous waterways. The region's aging bridges are being retrofitted for earthquake safety but remain at risk. Following the 2001 earthquake, engineers recommended tearing down the Alaska Way Viaduct (a tiered freeway rising high above Seattle's waterfront), because it cannot be brought into compliance with minimum safety standards. Still, the structure, though vulnerable, remains a major commuter artery. Multiple floating bridges in the area are vulnerable to earthquake or sabotage also.

Washington's large urban centers are clustered around the north–south Interstate 5 highway. Mountains to the east and west, forests, and extensive waterways isolate some rural communities from urban areas. These rural communities are subject to floods and forest fires, and their vulnerability is enhanced by their isolation.

VULNERABLE POPULATIONS

If disaster strikes, some population groups are at higher risk for injury. Particularly vulnerable are children, the elderly, those with serious chronic illness and immune suppression, refugees and others from diverse cultural and linguistic groups, the medically underserved, and the uninsured. Chou and colleagues found people with mental disorders, moderate physical disabilities, or who had been hospitalized just prior to earthquake were most vulnerable to death during a disaster in Taiwan [5]. The degree of vulnerability increased as socioeconomic status decreased.

Children

Children and infants represent at-risk populations in the face of any community-wide disaster. Children and infants must rely on adults for direction and the means to avoid or physically cope with natural disasters. Children and infants also must rely on adults for emotional support and guidance in the event of a disaster and must rely on adults to communicate their needs to the authorities and emergency personnel. In the event of a chemical or biological terrorist attack, children would be affected for several reasons. Physiologic factors conferring a great risk of adverse health outcomes in children include relatively higher minute ventilation, increased skin permeability, and a relatively large body surface area that can result in greater exposure. There is greater hypothermia risk if skin decontamination is not performed in a temperature-controlled environment. The preverbal child is more difficult to assess and triage. The protective clothing that health personnel must wear in the case of a chemical or biological event might frighten children. The same protective gear hampers dexterity, making it difficult to care for infants or small children. Potentially life-saving antimicrobial agents, antidotes, vaccines, and other pharmacologic agents have not been studied adequately in children, and, for many agents, pediatric doses were not established prior to 2000 [6].

Elderly persons

The elderly are vulnerable in the event of a disaster for some of the same reasons that children and infants are vulnerable. The elderly immune system is less competent and therefore more susceptible to various pathogens. The elderly are less agile and mobile and therefore more difficult to transport or evacuate in the face of disaster. The elderly are often subject to various chronic ailments that may be complicated or compounded by injuries, illnesses, or symptoms arising from a natural or intentional disaster. For example, chronic respiratory ailments common in the elderly make pathogens or chemical agents that affect the pulmonary system more likely to be associated with elevated morbidity and mortality. Also, various dementias, which are more prevalent in the elderly, can make it difficult for the elderly to communicate to emergency and health care workers or to follow instructions issued by authorities in a disaster. There also is some evidence that the elderly may be more susceptible to some mental disorders, such as depression, during or immediately following a large-scale terrorist event [7].

Patients with weakened immune systems

Those with weakened immune systems such as patients with HIV infection, cancer, those who have recently undergone organ transplantation, are more vulnerable to infection from biological agents [8]; the outcome in these individuals could be devastating. As people become ill with chronic diseases, they become increasingly vulnerable to infection. The risk of serious injury and infection in any disaster is intensified for people with chronic illnesses. Many chronic illnesses increase vulnerability to infection or injury. Patients with chronic obstructive pulmonary disease, asthma, emphysema, and other forms of chronic lung disease are more vulnerable than those with healthy lungs to damage caused by dust, smoke, and other inhaled substances resulting from explosions, fires, or other substances.

Culturally and linguistically diverse groups

Ethnically and culturally diverse groups are vulnerable in times of disaster. The linguistically diverse might not have access to mainstream communication channels and might not understand instructions related to safety and assistance. Culturally diverse groups similarly could lack understanding of available resources. Refugees who have escaped to the United States following traumatic events in their country of origin may be uniquely vulnerable to psychological trauma in association with a disaster. Prior violence exposure increases vulnerability to post-traumatic stress disorder, particularly among women [9,10].

Clinical exposures

Hanford Nuclear Reservation is located in a county where farming is a major industry. In the event of a nuclear disaster, those working in open fields are likely to receive more intense radiation exposure. Many farm workers are from migrant groups; thus it is important for nurses to be prepared to care for ethnically and culturally diverse patients and to work with diverse communities. Washington's Native Americans living along the Columbia River downstream from the Hanford site consume large quantities of fish from that river, another potential source of radiation exposure.

Some industrial regions are located disproportionately in poorer counties and neighborhoods, areas commonly medically underserved. Between 1890 and 1985, a copper smelter in western Washington released arsenic, lead, and other metallic pollutants into impoverished surrounding neighborhoods. Arsenic is a poison and a carcinogen [11]. The *Seattle Times* (March 22, 2001) reported fallout from the smelter had tainted the area [12]. Recently came the surprising revelation that sludge from the old plant was used to sandblast lead paint from a local water tower. This event demonstrates how easily human judgment may precipitate catastrophic events.

DEFINING AND VALIDATING COMPETENCIES

The disaster competency project used five types of potential threat, outlined in Table 1, as a framework. These potential threat categories were derived from literature on nursing disaster responsibilities, interpreted in the context of the regional need assessment, submitted for expert review and comment, then evaluated by nursing students and practicing nurses. It was acknowledged that an event could involve an agent or type of threat not emphasized in the resulting list of competencies. The educational programs built around the proposed competencies, however, would prepare nurses to improvise appropriately during disaster.

Table 1
Agents potentially causing regional disaster categories

Category of agent	Example in the Pacific Northwest
Prevailing or emerging infectious diseases occurring naturally or unintentionally (identified by state health department and/or the Centers for Disease Control and Prevention)	Foodborne illness (*Escherichia coli* O157:H7, *Salmonella*, *Campylobacter*, hepatitis A) Hantavirus
Toxic chemicals used or potentially abused in the region	Heavy metals (used in high technology industries) Chromic acid, cyanides, aluminum (fumes), and ammonia (used in aircraft manufacture) Chlorine gas (used in pulp and paper industry), Pesticides as noted on WA's PERT reports (Pesticide Exposure Report Tracking) (used in farming & forest management)
Radiological agent exposures	Accidental workplace exposures of Hanford Nuclear Reservation employees and environmental releases
Biological and chemical agents included in US Army handbook for medical management of chemical and biological casualties	Infectious agents (microorganisms causing anthrax, brucellosis, plague, Q-fever, tularemia, smallpox, viral encephalitis, and hemorrhagic fever), Nerve agents, cyanides, phosgene, vesicants (such as mustard gas), Bacteria-produced agents (staphylococcal enterotoxin B and botulinum toxin), Plant-derived toxin (ricin), Fungal metabolite (T-2 mycotoxin).
Natural occurrences likely to result in regional disaster	Earthquake Flood Fire Tsunami (on coastal region) Volcanic eruption

LITERATURE ON NURSING DISASTER COMPETENCIES

Disaster nursing competencies are not emphasized in nursing education, and there is scant literature on the topic. As noted by Gebbie and Quresh, training in basic disaster nursing competencies has not been a part of required undergraduate curricula at most United States nursing schools [13]. Until the Gebbie and Quresh publication in 2002, nursing competencies for emergency and disaster preparedness had not been defined for US nurses.

ENDORSEMENT OF COMPETENCIES BY EXPERTS

Health care institutions increasingly are aware of the need to improve disaster preparedness. Prompted by the events of Sept. 11, 2001, the Joint Commission on Accreditation of Hospitals (JCAHO) sent a special report to nearly 5000 hospitals and other health care facilities emphasizing the need for emergency preparedness. Standards for emergency management were revised and strengthened; included were standards for bioterrorism preparedness. These standards include identifying potential threats in the region, establishing decontamination procedures, community coordination of planning of alternative treatment facilities, and building relationships with other agencies. Hospitals will be cited for lack of compliance with the new standards. Weaknesses must be corrected within 6 months, or the institution faces potential loss of JCAHO accreditation. Hospitals must show evidence of planning and conducting drills, establishing relationships with community agencies, and implementing other strategies and training [14]. Hospitals, particularly those in remote and rural venues, have expressed a need for help with compliance.

NURSING EDUCATION DEFICITS

Nurses, working at the intersection of the public and the health care system, require preparation to respond effectively in catastrophic events, including terrorism, yet typically are not provided this preparation [15]. Nurses need to know strategies to recognize covert exposures in a population. Once a disaster is identified, it is typical that the incidence of psychological trauma exceeds the incidence of physical trauma. Nurses must understand the psychological responses to a disaster and work with patients and staff who may be experiencing psychological sequelae [16]. As vividly demonstrated in the sarin gas release in Tokyo subways, many secondary contamination casualties occurred among health care workers [17].

Nurses must know how to care for patients safely during a disaster. Nurses typically are involved in institutional and community planning of procedures and protocols for disasters; thus, they must know the current standards guiding institutional practice. They must know how to evaluate existing procedures and protocols, and often need skills in planning drills and practice events.

The Puget Sound area has many nursing education programs, but they lack disaster education content. There are seven baccalaureate nursing schools in the area (University of Washington-Seattle, University of Washington-Tacoma, University of Washington-Bothell, Seattle University, Seattle Pacific University, Pacific Lutheran University, and Northwest College). The required curricula for four of these schools were reviewed in 2002 and found to not have disaster content. Additionally, they did not offer elective content on the topic. The area's clinical facilities, nursing continuing education providers, and associate degree nursing programs do not fill this content void. Surveys conducted in two schools and two continuing education venues confirm the deficit in disaster content.

SURVEY RESPONSES

Students enrolled in baccalaureate nursing programs were surveyed in 2001 to determine their interest in the proposed disaster education content. The following results reflect interest in the proposed program. Fifty-four surveys were distributed to junior nursing students; 52 were returned. Of these, 50 (96%) juniors were somewhat or extremely interested in didactic disaster nursing content; 43 (83%) were somewhat or extremely interested in clinical applications of the disaster nursing content. Topics of primary interest were direct clinical care of afflicted individuals and safety of health care workers. Between 38 and 48 students (72% to 92%) said they were interested in subtopics such as chemical disasters and biological disasters. Fewer students (between 26 and 28 [50% to 54%]) were interested in health system topics such as collaborating with law enforcement and public health authorities, working with the Centers for Disease Control and Prevention (CDC), or communication procedures during a disaster.

Similarly, 31 surveys were distributed to senior nursing students. Of 29 respondents, 17 were extremely interested in attending an elective course; 11 were interested; one student was not interested (97% interested or extremely interested). As a group, the students indicated a strong preference for clinical topics.

Students at another western Washington school of nursing had similar interests. Forty-eight undergraduate students were surveyed in 2002. Of these, 46 (96%) were somewhat or extremely interested in disaster content; their preference for clinical topics paralleled the interests of the other nursing students.

Nurses enrolled in two continuing education offerings (one in an urban area, one in a rural area) were surveyed in 2001 to elicit their interest in disaster nursing content. Nurses (n = 33) attending a continuing education course in an urban area provided the following data. Twenty-nine nurses (88%) were somewhat or extremely interested in didactic disaster content; 18 (55%) were somewhat or extremely interested in clinical applications of the disaster nursing content. Eighteen nurses (55%) left their names with a request that they be contacted about future courses on the topic. Twenty-nine nurses (88%) said they would send employees to attend such a course. Topics of primary interest were similar to those of the students. Interest in direct clinical care of affected individuals prevailed over communication, collaboration, and community issues (29 nurses favored clinical topics; 16 endorsed health care system topics). There was a high level of interest in protecting the safety of health care workers. Most respondents preferred continuing education courses (n = 10) or Web-based offerings (n = 10), with eight nurses desiring a conventional academic course. Nurses (n = 13) attending a continuing education program in a rural community expressed intense interest in disaster nursing topics. All nurses surveyed (100%) were interested in attending courses related to disaster nursing and were interested in sending their employees. As with other groups, this group primarily was interested in clinical care issues. The rural nurses consistently requested that education be made available in their local community rather than require that they commute.

STATE AND REGIONAL IMPERATIVES

Improved response to public health emergencies and disasters is consistent with Washington State Health Department priorities, as set out in "Standards for Public Health in Washington State." Objective 8.1 is to "maintain and improve activities to prevent effects of well-known and familiar (microbial, chemical) hazards and...monitor developments related to emerging, often poorly understood hazards." Goal 8.11 is "...to reduce food-borne illness outbreaks caused by bacterial (eg, *E. coli, Salmonella,* and hepatitis A) viral, parasitic, or chemical agents transmitted by food [18]. The Pacific Northwest has experienced several catastrophes related to food-borne illness, intensifying awareness of this mechanism. An intentional salad bar tainting at 10 restaurants in The Dalles, Oregon, in 1984 by a religious cult resulted in 751 cases of salmonella illness. *E. coli* infections also have occurred in the Northwest. In 1993, 600 people were sickened, and four children died after eating contaminated beef at Jack-in-the-Box restaurants [19]. In 1996, a producer of unpasteurized apple juice was implicated in an outbreak of *E. coli* in the Pacific Northwest [20].

PROFESSIONAL NURSING MANDATE

Many professional organizations are focused on the need for improved disaster nursing preparation. The American Nurses Association (ANA) states on its bioterrorism and disaster response Web site, "as the nation copes with anthrax scares and concerns over future bioterrorist attacks, many nurses and other health care professionals have been forced to quickly learn about treating victims of bioterrorism, as well as to re-think their hospital and community disaster plans. ANA wants to ensure that registered nurses (RNs) will be able to respond effectively to these new types of emergencies and is working on several fronts to achieve this goal" [21].

The Emergency Nurses Association states, "on this day of critical nursing shortages and increased regulatory compliance issues, why should you focus any of your limited time on becoming educated on the topic of bioterrorism? By increasing awareness, knowing where your resources are, and following some basic infection control standards, the life you save may be your own. Early detection and identification can be the key to mobilizing national resources that are poised to combat the threat of an act of bioterrorism, and emergency nurses are on the front line of the war effort" [22].

The Association for Professionals in Infection Control and Epidemiology (APIC) made the following statement on preparedness. APIC "recognizes the importance of awareness and preparation for bioterrorism on the part of healthcare facilities. Hospitals and clinics may have the first opportunity to recognize and initiate a response to a bioterrorism-related outbreak. When developing the facility Bioterrorism Readiness Plan, provide for bioterrorism readiness education, including frank discussions of potential risks and plans for protecting healthcare providers" [23].

COMPETENCIES AND CONTENT

Entry-level disaster nursing competencies have been developed by the International Nursing Coalition for Mass Casualty Education and are available at http://www.aacn.nche.edu/Education/INCMCECompetencies.pdf [24]. INCMCE is a group of international nursing leaders and experts in education and mass casualty care. These competencies will be reviewed, revised, and updated each year.

BIOTERRORISM CURRICULUM ENHANCEMENT

A consortium of health science programs at the University of Washington, including the School of Nursing, received Health Resources and Services Administration (HRSA) funding for an Interdisciplinary Bioterrorism (BT) Curriculum Development project. This project is developing nursing discipline-specific BT content and content to teach students from multiple health science disciplines to work together in interdisciplinary teams. Both curricular approaches, discipline-specific and interdisciplinary, are important and complement one another. A goal of this project is to make the HRSA-funded curricular materials portable and available to nursing and health science programs throughout the country.

SUMMARY

Despite mitigation efforts, disasters are likely to increase in frequency and severity of impact because of increasing population density and other social and demographic trends. No region of the country is immune to the risk of major disaster; the risks emerge from the specific character of each community. Most nursing curricula currently lack disaster preparedness content. In this article, the vulnerabilities of the Pacific Northwest were analyzed. Undergraduate nursing students and practicing nurses from rural and urban communities expressed interest in disaster nursing content. These results and the core disaster nursing competencies for RNs have provided a framework to develop curricular elements and integrate those elements into nursing curricula. Next steps will include development of certificate programs so that nurses with expertise in disaster nursing can be credentialed for leadership.

References

[1] Veenema T, editor. Disaster nursing and emergency preparedness for chemical, biological, and radiological terrorism and other hazards. New York: Springer Publishing Company; 2003.

[2] Defensetech.org. Chemical "smoking guns" flame out—why? Available at: http://www.defensetech.org/archives/000339.html. Accessed January 18, 2005.

[3] Ellenhorn M. Medical toxicology: diagnosis and treatment of human poisoning. Baltimore (MD): Williams & Wilkins; 1996.

[4] Online PBS. Trail of a terrorist-other millennium attacks. Available at: http://www.pbs.org/wgbh/pages/frontline/shows/trail/inside/attacks.html. Accessed January 2001;18: 2005.

[5] Chou YJ, Huang N, Lee CH, et al. Who is at risk of death in an earthquake? Am J Epidemiol 2004;160(7):688–95.

[6] American Academy of Pediatrics Committee on Environmental Health and Committee on Infectious Diseases. Chemical and biological terrorism and its impact on children. Pediatrics 2000;105:662–70.

[7] Lomranz J, Hobfoll S, Johnson R, et al. A nation's response to attack: Israelis' depressive reactions to the Gulf War. J Trauma Stress 1994;7(1):59–73.

[8] Kaplan JE, Roselle G, Sepkowitz K. Opportunistic infections in immunodeficient populations. Emerg Infect Dis 1998;4(3):421–2.

[9] King DW, King LA, Foy DW, et al. Post-traumatic stress disorder in a national sample of female and male Vietnam veterans: risk factors, war-zone stressors, and resilience-recovery variables. J Abnorm Psychol 1999;108(1):164–70.

[10] Breslau N. Gender differences in trauma and posttraumatic stress disorder. J Gend Specif Med 2002;5(1):34–40.

[11] Agency for Toxic Substances and Disease Registry (ATSDR). ToxFAQs for arsenic. Available at: http://www.atsdr.cdc.gov/tfacts2.html. Accessed January 18, 2005.

[12] The Seattle Times. March 22, 2001.

[13] Gebbie KM, Qureshi K. Emergency and disaster preparedness: core competencies for nurses. Am J Nurs 2002;102(1):46–51.

[14] Joint Committee on Accreditation of Healthcare Organizations (JCAHO). Available at: http://www.jcrinc.com. Accessed January 18, 2005.

[15] Waeckerle JF, Seamans S, Whiteside M, et al. Executive summary: developing objectives, content, and competencies for the training of emergency medical technicians, emergency physicians, and emergency nurses to care for casualties resulting from nuclear, biological, or chemical incidents. Ann Emerg Med 2001;37(6):587–601.

[16] Beaton R, Murphy S. Psychosocial responses to biological and chemical terrorist threats and events: implications for the workplace and for occupational health nurses. AAOHN J 2002;50(4):182–9.

[17] Okumura T, Takasu N, Ishimatsu S, et al. Report on 640 victims of the Tokyo subway sarin attack. Ann Emerg Med 1996;28(2):129–35.

[18] Washington State Department of Health. Standards for public health in Washington State. Available at: http://www.doh.wa.gov/Standards/Default.htm#Contents. Accessed January 18, 2005.

[19] The News Tribune. Jack in the Box ignored safety rules. 1995.

[20] Cody SH, Glynn MK, Farrar JA, et al. An outbreak of Escherichia coli O157:H7 infection from unpasteurized commercial apple juice. Ann Intern Med 1999;130(4):202–9.

[21] American Nurses Association. Bioterrorism and disaster response Web site. Available at: http://www.nursingworld.org/news/disaster/. Accessed January 18, 2005.

[22] Stopford BM. Responding to the threat of bioterrorism: practical resources and references, and the importance of preparation. J Emerg Nurs 2001;127(5):471–5.

[23] English JF, Cundiff MY, Malone JD, et al. APIC Bioterrorism Task Force. Bioterrorism readiness plan: a template for healthcare facilities. Available at: http://www.cdc.gov/ncidod/hip/Bio/13apr99APIC-CDCBioterrorism.pdf. Accessed January 18, 2005.

[24] International Coalition of Mass Casualty Educators. Competencies for registered nurses. Available at: http://www.aacn.nche.edu/Education/INCMCECompetencies.pdf. Accessed January 18, 2005.

Nurs Clin N Am 40 (2005) 453–467

NURSING CLINICS
OF NORTH AMERICA

ELSEVIER
SAUNDERS

Disaster Competency Development and Integration in Nursing Education

Joan M. Stanley, PhD, RN, CRNP, FAAN[a,b,*]

[a]American Association of Colleges of Nursing, One Dupont Circle NW, Suite 530,
Washington, DC 20036, USA
[b]Faculty Practice Office, University of Maryland Hospital, 419 W. Redwood Street,
Baltimore, MD 21201, USA

Before Sept. 11, 2001, nurses were providing essential health services in response to mass casualty incidents (MCIs), including Hurricane Andrew, the Oklahoma City bombing, and the 2001 floods in Houston, Texas. Since Sept. 2001, however, the United States has undertaken a comprehensive reevaluation of its preparedness and the resources necessary to amass a response to critical events, particularly those posed by various forms of terrorism. The 2.7 million nurses registered to practice in the United States [1] represent a significant resource. This resource must be a core component of any national preparedness plan. To be effective, however, nursing must evaluate and enhance its own capabilities to respond to such events. Subsequently, nursing education must prepare nurses to fulfill this critical role.

Nurses are uniquely qualified to be early responders for MCIs or to deal with their long-term effects. They are expert in assessment skills, priority setting, and communication and collaboration. Additionally, they are prepared in an array of specialized areas from intensive care or trauma nursing, to public health nursing, to psychological–mental health nursing. Nurses are critical thinkers and can make decisions necessary in emergency situations. Nurses with advanced education and experience in trauma or critical care can fill more advanced triage, diagnostic, and treatment roles on the scene of an MCI. Because of the diverse educational background, experiences, and practice settings of nurses within the community and health care system, the potential roles of the professional nurse in an MCI may vary extensively.

To be an integral part of the community's plan for emergency preparedness in MCIs, nurses must have a basic level of education to appropriately respond and protect themselves and others, particularly during chemical, biological, radiologic, nuclear, and explosive (CBRNE) events. Not all nurses must be prepared to be first responders to CBRNE events. Every nurse, however, must

*American Association of Colleges of Nursing, One Dupont Circle NW, Suite 530, Washington, DC 20036, USA. E-mail address: jstanley@aacn.nche.edu

0029-6465/05/$ – see front matter
doi:10.1016/j.cnur.2005.04.009

have sufficient knowledge and skill to recognize the potential for an MCI, identify when such an incident may have occurred, know how to protect oneself, know how to provide immediate care for those individuals involved, recognize their own roles and limitations, and know where to seek additional information and resources. Nurses also must have sufficient knowledge to know when their own health and welfare may be in jeopardy and know how to protect themselves and others.

National nursing education standards and competencies do not mandate or recommend that all nurses be educated to respond to MCIs. Prior to the events of September 2001, nursing educators and organizations had begun to re-evaluate what nursing education's role should be in addressing the national and international response to MCIs.

NURSING EDUCATION'S ROLE IN DISASTER PREPAREDNESS

Nursing education's role is pivotal in ensuring that nursing as a discipline is prepared to meet its critical role in emergency preparedness plans. Successful implementation of this role depends on the participation and collaboration of education and professional organizations, accreditation and regulatory bodies or agencies, schools of nursing and individual faculty, and continuing education providers.

Broadly conceived, the roles of these four entities overlap and complement one another, producing change within the nursing profession. Increasing nurses' effectiveness for mass casualty preparedness highlights the necessary congruence within nursing.

THE INTERNATIONAL NURSING COALITION FOR MASS CASUALTY EDUCATION

Nursing education's role and preparation to respond to MCIs are reflected in the collaborative activities and goals of the International Nursing Coalition for Mass Casualty Education (INCMCE). This coalition, comprised of nursing organizations, specialty organizations, schools of nursing, regulators, accred-itors, and federal agencies, was spearheaded by the Department of Health and Human Services' Office of Emergency Preparedness (now Office of Emergency Response) and the Vanderbilt University School of Nursing. The goals of INCMCE include:

- Increasing the awareness and knowledge of all nurses about MCIs
- Influencing research efforts designed to improve nursing care and responses to MCIs
- Monitoring legislation and regulatory policies related to mass casualty education (MCE)
- Increasing effectiveness of all nurses responding to MCIs

Prior to September 2001, INCMCE had identified the first of these goals as the number one priority and issued a media release on nursing's important role in MCIs. After September 2001, the goals of the coalition were reversed, and the primary focus shifted to the effectiveness of nurses responding to MCIs.

ROLE OF NURSING EDUCATION AND PROFESSIONAL NURSING ORGANIZATIONS

The role of education and professional nursing organizations includes such activities as:

- Participation in the development and validation of core competencies
- Dissemination of competencies to members and other constituents
- Faculty development related to the core competencies and nursing education's role
- Development and assembling of resources to prepare nurses in the area of MCIs
- Provision of continuing education programs/materials for practicing nurses
- Seeking monies (eg, federal and state monies or foundational support) for the preparation of nurses and faculty
- Development and support of a research framework related to MCIs

ROLE OF ACCREDITATION AND REGULATORY AGENCIES

The role of specialty nursing accreditation bodies, such as the Commission on Collegiate Nursing Education (CCNE) and the National League for Nursing Accrediting Commission (NLNAC), includes such activities as:

- Participation in the development and validation of core competencies
- Determining whether the MCI competencies should be required of and documented by a program or school to receive accreditation
- Determining whether MCI content in any form should be mandated for inclusion in a nursing program

The Joint Commission on Accreditation of Healthcare Organizations (JCAHO) mandates specific areas in which all health care institutions must ensure that employees are prepared. As part of a national emergency preparedness plan, JCAHO could mandate that health care institutions be required to document the competence of all employed registered nurses (RNs) and other health professionals regarding their ability to appropriately respond to MCIs. After September 2001, JCAHO modified its accreditation standards for hospitals to include requirements regarding emergency planning, exercises, and training [2].

State boards of nursing maintain a nursing education program review function, some to a greater degree than others. In establishing criteria for licensure within the state, a state board of nursing could mandate that a candidate for a registered nurse license graduate from a program that includes MCI content or has documented competence regarding MCI response. Several state boards also mandate continuing education credits for licensure renewal. A certification or continuing education program in mass casualty response could be developed and required for license renewal. The National Council

Licensure Examination (NCLEX) administered by the National Council of State Boards of Nursing (NCSBN) is based on role delineation studies of practicing nurses. As the role of the practicing nurse evolves to include preparation for emergency preparedness, MCI content could be included in the national licensure examination.

SCHOOLS OF NURSING AND FACULTY ROLES

Schools of nursing and nursing faculty play critical roles in preparing nurses for emergency preparedness and response. Specific activities and roles include:

- Participation in the development and validation of core competencies
- Curriculum development or redesign to include content and clinical experiences related to MCIs
- Development and maintenance of faculty expertise and competence
- Assessment of the competence of graduates
- Development of teaching resources and materials
- Design and implementation of research related to MCIs and improving nursing care and responses in MCIs

ROLE OF CONTINUING EDUCATION PROVIDERS

Although similar to that of nursing faculty and frequently dependent upon regulatory and accreditation standards, continuing education providers have a critical role in educating RNs and assuring effective response to MCIs. Specifically, the role of continuing education providers includes:

- Development of continuing education modules or courses in various formats, including traditional classroom and Web-based formats
- Dissemination of learning resources and materials
- Education of RNs practicing in varied settings and with very diverse education and practice backgrounds

INCREASING EFFECTIVENESS OF RESPONSES TO MASS CASUALTY INCIDENTS

Immediately after September 2001, increasing the effectiveness of all nurses in responding to MCIs became the primary focus of INCMCE. Nursing education standards have not mandated or recommended that nurses graduating from entry-level nursing programs or advanced practice nursing programs receive preparation related to MCIs. More recently however, many nursing schools have been evaluating and augmenting their curricula related to disaster response and care of mass casualties. Likewise, most health care institutions previously did not recognize the need or importance of requiring nurses and other health care professionals to receive training related to MCIs or had trained only a select group as part of an emergency response team. To ensure that nurses are prepared to respond appropriately and safely to MCIs and to assist nursing schools and continuing education providers to meet this challenge, INCMCE developed a set of core competencies related to mass casualty incidents for all entry-level nurses.

PROCESS TO DEVELOP MASS CASUALTY EDUCATION NURSING COMPETENCIES

Two phases, an internal and an external review phase, were used for the development of consensus-based competencies for MCE of all nurses. A subcommittee of INCMCE, comprised of representatives of schools of nursing and national nursing education and accreditation organizations, was identified to accomplish this task. Competencies for MCE were developed previously for various groups of health care professionals. Therefore, prior to developing a set of MCE nursing competencies, existing educational curricula and sets of competencies were reviewed and evaluated. The recommendations and competencies developed by the subcommittee were based heavily on the competencies delineated by other health profession groups, including the Task Force of Health Care and Emergency Services Professionals [3]; Association of State and Territorial Directors of Nursing [4]; Center for Health Policy, Columbia School of Nursing [5]; University of Ulster, University of Glamorgan School of Health Sciences School of Nursing [6]; and the Uniformed Services University of the Health Sciences Graduate School of Nursing (Faye G. Abdellah, personal communication, 2001).

Following the initial review and evaluation of these existing health profession documents, a set of entry-level or basic competencies was developed by the subcommittee and presented to the larger coalition. During this initial internal phase, the coalition and subcommittee had several opportunities to provide input and recommend revisions. Upon completion of this first phase, phase two or the external review phase involved a validation panel comprised of a larger group of representatives from nursing practice, education, accreditation, and certification. Validation panel members reviewed the competencies to assess their relevance, specificity, and comprehensiveness for entry-level nursing.

Using the previously developed competency validation tool and process [7], participants on the validation panel were asked to review systematically each individual competency according to the following criteria:

- Relevance. Is the competency necessary? (yes, no, or do not know)
- Specificity. Is the competency stated specifically and clearly? (yes, no, do not know, and suggested rewording)
- Comprehensiveness. In your opinion, if there is any aspect of general nursing knowledge, skill, or personal attributes missing? (Please enter those new competencies.)

Based on feedback from the validation panel, a national, consensus-based set of educational competencies for RNs responding to MCIs was endorsed by INCMCE [8].

The dissemination and implementation of these national consensus-based competencies is ongoing. One of the critical steps in the implementation of the competencies and the effective preparation of nurses is integrating content and skills into the nursing curriculum.

MASS CASUALTY EDUCATION COMPETENCIES FOR ALL NURSES

What is meant by all nurses? All practicing nurses? All licensed RNs? All retired nurses? Student nurses? Nurses practicing in all settings and specialty areas? These are some of the questions with which INCMCE members struggled. A general consensus among coalition members prevailed: that all RNs currently licensed to practice and all nurses educated from now on should have some basic level of knowledge and skill related to MCIs. This very broad definition of all nurses is the ultimate target for preparing nurses with competence in MCI preparedness and response.

To facilitate the integration of the MCE competencies into the nursing curricula, an existing nursing curriculum framework was used as a basis for the development of the competencies. *The Essentials of Baccalaureate Education for Professional Nursing Practice* [9] provides a framework for baccalaureate nursing curricula. The essentials of professional nursing education include five key components: liberal education, professional values, core competencies, core knowledge, and role development. Using this framework, the three components addressed by the MCE document are core competencies, core knowledge, and role development.

COMPETENCY FRAMEWORK

The American Association of Colleges of Nursing (AACN) essentials [9] were used as a framework for delineating outcome competencies related to MCIs expected of all RNs. To highlight the knowledge and skill level expected of all nurses in the future, examples of the MCI competencies embedded within the essentials framework are presented in Appendix 1.

CORE COMPETENCIES

The nursing MCI competencies related to professional role development are not differentiated by specific roles, such as provider of care, designer/manager/coordinator of care, or member of a profession. Areas of competence encompass all three critical nursing roles. Several examples of the competencies are listed in Box 1.

INTEGRATING MASS CASUALTY EDUCATION INTO THE NURSING CURRICULUM

Sixty-four competencies are delineated in the INCMCE *Educational Competencies for Registered Nurses Responding to Mass Casualty Incidents* [8]. These national consensus-based competencies apply to all professional RN roles and practice settings, and are intended to describe entry-level practice. All nurses from novice to expert should have a basic knowledge and ability to respond to MCIs independent of their education and practice experience. The individual

Box 1: Mass casualty incident competencies concerning professional role development [8]

Identify the most appropriate or most likely health care role for oneself during an MCI.

Describe the nursing roles in MCIs

- Researcher
- Investigator/epidemiologist
- EMT or first responder
- Direct care provider, generalist nurse
- Direct care provider, advanced practice nurse (APN)
- Director/coordinator of care in hospital/nurse administrator or emergency department nurse manager
- Onsite coordinator of care/incident commander
- Onsite director of care management
- Information provider or educator, particularly the role of the generalist nurse
- Mental health counselor
- Member of planning response team
- Member of community assessment team
- Manager or coordinator of shelter
- Member of decontamination team
- Triage officer

Identify the limits to one's own knowledge/skills/abilities/authority related to MCIs.

Recognize the importance of maintaining one's expertise and knowledge in this area of practice and of participating in regular emergency response drills.

competencies are intentionally general and must be interpreted in relation to the functional role of an individual nurse within an agency or community. Competencies will be applied to practice in differing ways depending on the specific roles and responsibilities the nurse performs within the health care system or community. Therefore, the dilemma for nursing educators is to determine how can graduates be prepared with this knowledge and skill set? And what content and experiences are already being taught, and what needs to be added or augmented?

Much of the knowledge and experiences underpinning the competencies related to appropriate and timely response to MCIs are basic to nursing practice. Therefore, most of the principles and information necessary for the development of competence in these areas are included in all basic nursing education programs to some degree. Until the past several years, however, most nursing educators, or the population in general, did not focus on emergency preparedness and the role nurses should play. Therefore, the context in which these MCI competencies may be taught and utilized could vary dramatically.

An overall assessment of the existing curriculum is recommended prior to adding any additional content or clinical experiences. Many schools have used curriculum mapping not only for identifying content related to MCE, but also for any general knowledge area that is threaded throughout the curriculum. Frequently what occurs is new content is added to one or two courses without evaluating how this content builds upon or supports content and experiences throughout the remaining curriculum. Critical questions that nursing educators must ask are:

- What content and experiences are already included in the curriculum that address the MCI competencies?
- What basic content or principles that are already being taught can be reframed in order to redirect or refocus critical thinking and application surrounding this content?
- What content and experiences, already included in the curriculum, can be enhanced or supplemented to prepare graduates with the necessary competence related to MCIs?
- What additional content and experiences specific to emergency preparedness and MCI response need to be added to the curriculum?
- What pedagogical techniques can be used best for preparing graduates with these competencies?
- What resources are available to teach this content?
- How can the competence of graduates related to MCI preparedness be assessed?
- How best can we evaluate the curriculum and teaching methodologies used to achieve these outcomes?

INTEGRATING MASS CASUALTY INCIDENT CONTENT INTO NURSING COURSES

Much of the knowledge and experiences underpinning the MCI competencies are basic to nursing practice and already are included in the nursing curriculum. The competencies transcend all essential components of nursing education. New ways of presenting or re-emphasizing existing content or principles throughout the entire curriculum to stimulate critical thinking and the development of new skills related to MCIs is necessary. New case studies, new teaching–learning modules, simulations, small group discussions, and community-based experiences are among the pedagogies that could be used to achieve this goal. Examples of how content could be integrated throughout a typical nursing curriculum are outlined in Box 2. This is not intended to be a definitive outline for the placement or inclusion of all MCI content within the nursing curriculum. Rather it is intended as a starting point for evaluating and planning MCI curriculum.

The Federal Emergency Management Agency (FEMA) and other government agencies provide courses and training opportunities for field experiences

Box 2: Ways to integrate mass casualty incident content

Physical assessment course
History taking to elicit information about possible exposure to CBRNE agents, including place of employment, living, and recreation; recent travel; unexplained or vague symptoms; illness of family members, friends, and coworkers

Focused history taking to assess potential exposure to CBRNE, including signs and symptoms related to specific body systems

- Skin. Rashes, burns from radiation or chemical burns, or lesions
- Gastrointestinal system, Nausea, vomiting, or diarrhea
- Respiratory system. Cough or shortness of breath
- General. Elevated temperature and other potential changes in vital signs
- Neurological. Unexplained neurological changes, symptoms of intracranial pressure, or other symptoms of trauma
- Eye. Pain or changes in vision related to foreign bodies or chemical exposures.

Perform an age-appropriate assessment of a patient exposed to various CBRNE agents.

Advanced clinical skills laboratory course
Practice donning and working in personal protective equipment (PPE).

Discuss and practice decontamination principles and exercises in a health care institution and in other settings.

Demonstrate the use of various types of communication equipment used in the field during an MCI.

Practice basic therapeutic interventions (eg, basic first aid skills, oxygen administration and ventilation techniques, lavage techniques, and initial wound care) in a community setting with limited equipment and supplies.

Demonstrate principles of patient safety during transport through splinting, immobilizations, and monitoring.

Pathophysiology course
Neurological system. Discuss signs and symptoms of poisonous gas exposure and other agents and potential effects of other forms of trauma (eg, increased intracranial pressure).

Respiratory system. Discuss signs and symptoms, differential diagnosis of biologic and chemical agents that can be weaponized, such as anthrax.

Cardiovascular system. Discuss the signs and symptoms of biologic and chemical agent exposure and the impact on the cardiovascular system.

Infectious diseases. Discuss newly emerging infectious agents such as Severe Acute Respiratory Syndrome, signs and symptoms, detection and control.

Adult health course
When discussing principles of infection control and isolation techniques, introduce a scenario that encompasses multiple individuals, various biologic agents, and various settings.

Care of children course
Discuss the potential short- and long-term effects of an MCI on children of various ages, ethnicities, and cultures.

Discuss appropriate coping strategies that could be implemented with a group of school-aged children.

Mental health nursing course
Include content related to post-traumatic stress disorder and acute anxiety disorder and relate to responses to MCIs.

Include a discussion of group therapy application or measures for stress reduction for large groups/communities.

Identify all who may need mental health counseling during and after a disaster, including health care workers, the injured, family members, community members, and the nation. Discuss appropriate resources for referring and treating these various groups.

Practice principles of risk communication to groups and individuals affected by exposure during an MCI.

Discuss the cultural, spiritual, and social issues that may affect an individual's response to an MCI.

Community health nursing course
As part of a community assessment, identify possible threats and their potential impact on the health care system and community at large in a specified locale or geographic area.

Identify community health issues related to limiting exposure to selected MCI agents; water, air, and food supply contamination; and shelter and protection of displaced persons in the community.

Describe the local chain of command and management system for emergency response during an MCI in a specific community or region.

Discuss how agencies/resources are coordinated and the role(s) of each in an MCI.

Include a discussion and simulation of communication networks that are essential for smooth delivery of care and control of panic.

Review and discuss the identified community disaster plan for local community or region. Identify individual roles for nurses. Identify one's own potential role within the community disaster plan.

Health care systems and organizations
Review and discuss at least one health care institution's disaster plan with focus on the various roles (or potential roles) of nurses.

Identify and discuss the impact various types of MCIs potentially would have on the health care institution(s) in the local community, including personnel, pharmaceuticals, and medical supplies.

Ethics
In an interprofessional seminar, discuss issues related to abandonment of patients; roles and responsibilities assumed by volunteer efforts; rights of individuals to refuse care; allocation of limited resources; and rights and responsibilities of health care providers in MCIs.

When discussing end-of-life care, discuss the ethical, legal, psychological, and cultural considerations when dealing with the dying or handling and storage of human remains in an MCI.

Use the American Nurse's Association Position Statement on Work Release During a Disaster: Guidelines for Employers [10] as a basis for discussion on responsibilities of nurses and other health care providers during an MCI, or on potential roles of nurses during an MCI.

related to CRBNE responses and disaster drills. Schools of nursing could collaborate with the local Emergency Medical Service or other agency to schedule their nursing students to participate in a disaster field experience. This exercise could be incorporated into the curriculum as a 1-week clinical experience. It also is recommended that all RNs participate in biannual emergency response drills organized through the Office of Emergency Preparedness.

FUTURE WORK AND CHALLENGES

The nursing community has recognized the potential impact that nurses can and should make in emergency preparedness and response. Other health care providers and federal, state, and local agencies are following the INCMCE lead in developing provider competencies, developing learning resources, and ensuring that nurses are prepared and a central component of any disaster response plan.

The INCMCE, nursing organizations, and schools face additional challenges in assuring an adequately prepared nursing workforce. Specialized MCI competencies should be developed for APNs and nurses in specialized areas of practice. APN competencies that address the higher-level triage, diagnostic, and treatment capabilities of the APN, inter-professional collaboration, health policy, and the broad systems focus the APN brings to the health care arena would further define the APN as a significant resource in emergency preparedness. In addition, the development of MCI competencies and the delineation of roles for other nursing specialties, such as administration, community health, critical care, and school health, would assist government and health care planners in appropriately using nurses in emergency response plans.

Faculty development in the area of MCE is an immediate need. As government agencies and health care institutions broaden the expectations and requirements related to emergency preparedness and response, there will be a growing demand for continuing education providers and nursing faculty with the necessary MCI expertise.

The need for quality resources for group and individual learning related to MCIs and emergency preparedness presents another immediate challenge for nursing education. Immediately after September 2001, many Web sites, reports, and articles appeared. Faculties attempting to develop appropriate programming or curricula for nurses or other health professionals were overwhelmed. Resources, including learning/teaching modules, are being developed for nurses and other health care professionals. Veenema has developed a companion curriculum guide for her text on disaster nursing [11]. In addition, a full on-line course and curriculum are being developed. An on-line curriculum also is being developed at the Vanderbilt University School of Nursing. Other teaching modules and health profession curricula are being developed through 2003 Health Resources and Services Administration cooperative agreements.

Finally, a research framework that addresses nursing roles in MCIs, appropriate responses, preparedness, and outcomes should be developed. Because of the nature of MCIs and the need for an interprofessional response, a collaborative research framework and approach would seem to address this pressing need best.

SUMMARY

Ensuring that nursing as a profession is prepared to meet the country's need for emergency preparedness requires the collaborative effort of all nursing education as broadly described. Schools of nursing and individual faculty have a particularly challenging task of ensuring that all future nursing graduates have basic knowledge and skills related to MCIs. The INCMCE has developed a set of national consensus-based competencies that provide a framework for MCI education. Educating 2.7 million nurses and all future nurses regarding MCIs is an unheralded feat; however, nurses, because of their unique nursing education and perspective practicing in multiple roles and settings, provide an unduplicated resource for mass casualty preparedness and response.

APPENDIX 1. EXAMPLES OF THE EDUCATIONAL COMPETENCIES FOR REGISTERED NURSES RELATED TO MASS CASUALTY INCIDENTS [8]

Core competencies

  I. Critical thinking
    A. Use an ethical and nationally approved framework to support decision-making and prioritizing needed in disaster situations.
    B. Use clinical judgment and decision-making skills in assessing the potential for appropriate, timely individual care during an MCI.
  II. Assessment
    A. General
      • Assess the safety issues for self, the response team, and victims in any given response situation, in collaboration with the incident response team.
      • Identify possible indicators of a mass exposure (ie, clustering of individuals with the same symptoms).
      • Describe the essential elements included in an MCI scene assessment.
    B. Specific
      • Conduct a focused health history to assess potential exposures to CBRNE agents.
      • Assess the immediate psychological response of the individual, family, or community following an MCI.
      • Perform an age-appropriate health assessment, including:
        1. Airway and respiratory assessment
        2. Cardiovascular assessment, including vital signs and monitoring for signs of shock

3. Integumentary assessment, particularly a wound, burn, and rash assessment
4. Pain assessment
5. Injury assessment from head to toe
6. Gastrointestinal assessment, including specimen collection
7. Basic neurological assessment
8. Musculoskeletal assessment
9. Mental status, spiritual, and emotional assessment

III. Technical skills
A. Demonstrate safe administration of medications, particularly vasoactive and analgesic agent, by oral (PO), subcutaneous (SQ), intramuscular (IM), and intravenous (IV) administration routes.
B. Demonstrate the safe administration of immunizations, including smallpox vaccination.
C. Assess the need for and initiate the appropriate CBRNE isolation and decontamination procedures available, ensuring that all parties understand the need.
D. Demonstrate knowledge and skill related to personal protection and safety, including the use PPE for Level B and C protections and respiratory protection.
E. Demonstrate the ability to maintain patient safety during transport through splinting, immobilization, monitoring, and therapeutic interventions.

IV. Communication
A. Describe the local chain of command and management system for emergency response during an MCI.
B. Identify one's own role in the emergency response plan for the place of employment.
C. Demonstrate appropriate emergency documentation of assessments, interventions, nursing actions, and outcomes during and after an MCI.
D. Identify appropriate resources for referring requests from patients, media, or others for information regarding MCIs.
E. Describe appropriate coping strategies to manage self and others.
F. Core competencies
I. Health promotion, risk reduction, and disease prevention
A. Identify possible threats and their potential impact on the general public, emergency medical system, and the health care community.
B. Describe community health issues related to MCI events, specifically limiting exposure to selected agents; contamination of water, air, and food supplies; and shelter and protection of displaced persons.
II. Health care systems and policy
A. Define and distinguish the terms disaster and MCI in relation to other major incidents or emergency situations.
B. Define relevant terminology, including:
1. CBRNE
2. Weapons of mass destruction (WMD)
3. Triage
4. Chain of command and management system for emergency response
5. PPE

6. Scene assessment
7. Comprehensive emergency management
C. Describe the legal authority of public health agencies to take action to protect the community from threats, including isolation, quarantine, and required reporting and documentation.
D. Recognize the impact MCIs may have on access to resources and identify how to access additional resources (eg, pharmaceuticals and medical supplies).
III. Illness and disease management
A. Discuss the differences/similarities between an intentional biological attack and that of a natural disease outbreak.
B. Describe, using an interdisciplinary approach, the short- and long-term effects of physical and psychological symptoms related to disease and treatment secondary to MCIs.
IV. Information and health care technologies
A. Describe the use of emergency communication equipment that must be used in a MCI response.
B. Discuss the principles of containment and decontamination.
C. Describe how nursing skills may have to be adapted while wearing PPE.
V. Ethics
A. Identify and discuss ethical issues related to MCI events, including:
1. Rights and responsibilities of health care providers in MCIs (eg, refusing to go to work or report for duty or refusal of vaccines)
2. Need to protect the public versus an individual's right for autonomy (eg, right to leave the scene after contamination)
3. Right of the individual to refuse care, informed consent
4. Allocation of limited resources
5. Confidentiality of information related to individuals and national security
6. Use of public health authority to restrict individual activities, requiring reporting from health professionals, and collaborating with law enforcement
B. Describe the ethical, legal, psychological, and cultural considerations when dealing with the dying and/or the handling and storage of human remains in an MCI.
C. Identify and discuss legal and regulatory issues related to:
1. Abandonment of patients
2. Response to an MCI and one's position of employment
3. Various roles and responsibilities assumed by volunteer efforts
VI. Human diversity
A. Discuss the cultural, spiritual, and social issues that may affect an individual's response to an MCI.
B. Discuss the diversity of emotional, psychosocial and socio–cultural responses to terrorism or the threat of terrorism to one's self and others.

- A seventh area of core knowledge, Global Health Care, is included in the AACN Essentials document. Through the consensus-building process to develop a set of national nursing MCI competencies, no competencies were identified or categorized under this core knowledge area. Many of the MCI competencies, however, overlap areas of content and skill and could be identified under several areas of core competence, core knowledge, or professional development.

References

[1] Spratley E, Johnson A, Sochalski J, et al. The registered nurse population findings from the national sample survey of registered nurses. Washington (DC): U S Department of Health and Human Services, Health Resources and Services Administration, Bureau of Health Professions, Division of Nursing; 2000.

[2] Joint Commission on Accreditation of Healthcare Organizations. Special issue. Joint Commission Perspectives 2001;21(12):1–23. Available at: jcrinc.com/docviewer.aspx. Accessed June 1, 2005.

[3] Task Force of Health Care and Emergency Services Professionals on Preparedness for Nuclear, Biological, and Chemical Incidents. Final report: developing objectives, content, and competencies for the training of emergency medical technicians, emergency physicians, and emergency nurses to care for casualties resulting from nuclear, biological, or chemical (NBC) incidents (Contract No. 282-98-0037). Washington (DC): Department of Health and Human Services and American College of Emergency Physicians; 2001.

[4] Association of State and Territorial Directors of Nursing. Position paper: public health nurses' vital role in emergency preparedness and response. Atlanta (GA): Association of State and Territorial Directors of Nursing; 2002.

[5] Center for Health Policy. Columbia University School of Nursing. Core public health worker competencies for emergency preparedness and response. Atlanta (GA): Centers for Disease Control and Prevention; 2001.

[6] University of Ulster, University of Glamorgan School of Health Sciences School of Nursing. Course document for postgraduate diploma/MSc in disaster relief nursing for entry September 1999. Ulster (UK): University of Ulster; 1998.

[7] National Organization of Nurse Practitioner Faculties & American Association of Colleges of Nursing. Nurse practitioner primary care competencies in specialty areas: adult, family, gerontological, pediatric, and women's health. Rockville (MD): Department of Health and Human Services, Health Resources and Services Administration, Bureau of Health Professions, Division of Nursing; 2002.

[8] International Nursing Coalition for Mass Casualty Education. Educational competencies for registered nurses responding to mass casualty incidents. Available at: http://www.aacn.nche.edu/Education/pdf/INCMCECompetencies.pdf. Accessed May 31, 2005.

[9] American Association of Colleges of Nursing. The essentials of baccalaureate education for professional nursing practice. Washington (DC): American Association of Colleges of Nursing; 1998.

[10] American Nurses Association. Position Statement on work release during a disaster: guidelines for employers. Adopted by the ANA Board of Directors. Effective June 24, 2002. Available at: http://www.nursingworld.org/readroom/position/social/scwrkrel.htm. Accessed May 31, 2005.

[11] Veenema TG, editor. Disaster nursing and emergency preparedness for chemical, biological and radiological terrorism and other hazards. New York, NY: Springer Publishing Company; 2003.

Nurs Clin N Am 40 (2005) 469–479

NURSING CLINICS
OF NORTH AMERICA

A National Curriculum for Nurses in Emergency Preparedness and Response

Elizabeth E. Weiner, PhD, RN, BC, FAAN

International Nursing Coalition for Mass Casualty Education, Vanderbilt University School of Nursing, 461 21st Avenue South, Nashville, TN 37240, USA

The growing number of terror attacks has caused the United States to recognize real threats in the environment. A more reasonable approach has been in the recent movement to plan and improve responses to various hazards (thus the term "all hazards" approach). Some nurses have had community health education related to natural disasters. Most have not, however, been educated about biological, chemical, nuclear, explosive, or radiological hazards. Biological hazards place health care providers in the position of being first responders or first receivers. Traditionally, first responders have been the police, firefighters, and emergency medical technicians who respond on the scene. In a covert biological event, victims will appear first in an emergency department (ED), clinic, or school health setting. Health care professionals need to be able to identify symptoms, data patterns, and other irregularities. If they fail to recognize or report significant events, an attack could go unrecognized until it is too late.

THE AMERICAN COLLEGE OF EMERGENCY PHYSICIANS TASK FORCE

Because the ED most likely would receive the first victims of a bioterrorism, chemical, or nuclear attack, it is no surprise that the first needs assessment and curricular review centered on the ED. The American College of Emergency Physicians (ACEP) formed a nuclear, biological and chemical task force to evaluate the status of bioterrorism training in the United States, identify barriers to this training, and offer recommendations for effective education [1]. As a result, content needs were addressed for emergency nurses, physicians, and emergency medical technicians. The US Department of Health and Human Services (DHHS)' Office of Emergency Preparedness (now the Office of Emergency Response) sponsored the task force.

This work was supported by contracts from the Department of Health and Human Services.

E-mail address: betsy.weiner@vanderbilt.edu

During their analysis, the task force focused on a definition of the problem that would result in specific recommendations. They produced a description of the target audiences/learners, an outline of the content that learners should be taught with specific objectives that indicate what learners must know and be able to do, clarification of barriers, and a review of existing educational materials.

Specific methods were used to describe the targeted audiences, including group interactions, interviews, review of materials, and agreement by the task force. The task force determined the relative similarities and differences among the groups in several areas. Based on the information gathered, a subject matter analysis was accomplished through interviews with task force members and other subject matter experts recommended by the task force. Additional detail was added after reviewing selected articles and other existing subject matter material. The content was organized into three proficiency categories: awareness, performance, and planning. Objectives for each of these categories then were developed.

A formal curriculum review was undertaken. The focus of each review was to assess current educational efforts regarding specific weapons of mass destruction (WMD) and to determine how to best integrate that content into the educational programs designed for each audience. The task force concluded, "from initial nurse education through the educational path selected to reach the emergency nursing specialty, emergency nurses are provided no course work specific to WMD incidents" [1].

BARRIERS TO IMPLEMENTATION

Barriers were identified that would make integration of this content into nursing school curricula difficult. These include:

- Lack of funding for developing comprehensive WMD content for nursing school or for continuing education materials/courses, including research, writing, material development, faculty development, and pilot testing
- Lack of a national clearing house or repository for collection of related knowledge and skills currently being developed to ensure consistency and quality and minimize redundancy of effort
- Difficulty procuring adequate expertise to work on the development of curricula and course materials and to oversee content development, management, and revision
- Lack of perception by hospital leadership that this type of training is a top priority

The ACEP report was viewed as a starting point for mass casualty education. Critics were quick to point out that the findings of the report focused specifically on EDs and were not therefore generalizable to other areas. In addition, the review focused on nuclear, biological and chemical WMDs rather than a broader view including explosive, radiological, or natural causes of events.

INITIAL PUBLIC HEALTH WORKFORCE COMPETENCY DEVELOPMENT

While the ACEP Report was being prepared, another effort was underway. Kristine M. Gebbie, RN, DrPH, examined whether the nation's public health workforce was ready to respond to emergencies. Gebbie published the first version of competencies for public health workers in 2001 [2]. Some of the competencies were applicable to every worker; others were specific to workers in administrative, professional, technical, or support positions. This work later was expanded to encompass specific bioterrorism competencies and to include competencies for more job categories [3]. The document notes that "the application of any competency is always within the context of both agency and jurisdictional plans" [3]. The type of emergency and the emergency response plan for each jurisdiction also determine whether a public health agency is in the lead position, in a collaborative role, or in a secondary/supportive role. The same is true for other organizations that comprise an emergency response team.

THE INTERNATIONAL NURSING COALITION FOR MASS CASUALTY EDUCATION

Captain Veronica Stephens of the DHHS Office of Emergency Preparedness reviewed the ACEP report and the public health competencies. She wanted to see the formation of an organization to provide leadership and support for nurses in the area of mass casualty education. A partnership was developed with the Vanderbilt University School of Nursing because of the efforts of Dean Colleen Conway-Welch. The partnership grew to be the International Nursing Coalition for Mass Casualty Education (INCMCE). The group first met in March 2001 with sponsorship from DHHS.

The International Nursing Coalition for Mass Casualty Education is an international coalition consisting of organizational representatives of schools of nursing, nursing accrediting bodies, nursing specialty organizations, and government agencies interested in promoting mass casualty education for nurses. The vision of the organization is to be the point of influence for public policy that impacts the welfare of the public through nursing practice, education, research, and regulation for mass casualty incidents (MCIs). The mission is to assure a competent nurse workforce to respond to MCIs. A strategic plan has been developed in the priority areas of awareness, response, and research.

INTERNATIONAL FOCUS

One of the reasons INCMCE was established as an international group was to take advantage of lessons learned from international colleagues. The first nursing program in disaster response was established at the University of Ulster, Northern Ireland [10]. The Japanese Nursing Disaster Society is an INCMCE member, and that organization already has provided insight into lessons learned from the Kobe earthquake and other emergencies such as tsunamis and the Tokyo sarin gas episode. Nurses from Israel also have been willing to share their expertise in providing education in emergency preparedness and response to their nurses.

International Nursing Coalition for Mass Casualty Education members recognized that curriculum content in nursing programs never had been validated, so a survey was prepared by an INCMCE task force. In conjunction with the National League for Nursing, an online curricular survey was sent to all deans and directors of nursing programs in the United States in 2003. The results of this survey not only provide baseline data in relation to what nursing programs are teaching at all levels in emergency response, but it will be the source of annual data collection over 5 years.

THE INTERNATIONAL NURSING COALITION FOR MASS CASUALTY EDUCATION SURVEY OF NURSING PROGRAMS' CONTENT

Over 300 schools of nursing representing 455 different nursing programs (from LPN/LVN through doctorate) responded to the survey. Most striking was the finding that 75% of the respondents felt that faculty were not at all prepared or poorly prepared to teach disaster preparedness content.

During the 2000–2001 school year, only 22% (N = 107) of the schools of nursing in the survey offered disaster preparedness content, with natural disasters receiving the greatest emphasis (28% of programs). During the 2001–2002 school year, the percentage of nursing schools offering some disaster preparedness content rose to 39%, again with an emphasis on natural disaster. Disasters related to biological and chemical agents, however, began receiving more emphasis. It was not until this last academic year that content related to biological agents occurred more frequently than content related to natural disasters, and content related to chemical agents increased significantly. It should be noted that content related to nuclear, radiological, and explosive agents has lagged behind in all 3 academic years Fig. 1.

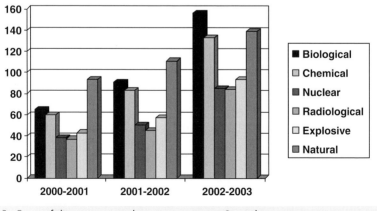

Fig. 1. Focus of disaster preparedness content across 3 academic years.

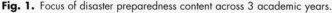

Although biological and chemical agents have received increasing emphasis in disaster preparedness content in nursing programs, the total contact hours over the 3 years has not changed significantly. The average number of contact hours in disaster preparedness content is approximately 4 hours (means ranged from 3.9 from 2000 to 2001 to 4.2 from 2002 to 2003). Most respondents were using Web sites (50%) and journal articles (45.8%) to provide content in disaster preparedness.

Most of the nursing programs relied on lectures (52% to 58%) to deliver disaster preparedness content, with other delivery modalities such as seminars, field experiences, independent study, or online classes used less frequently. Fewer than 17% of respondents indicated that they used these other modalities.

Survey respondents overwhelmingly indicated that a curriculum plan in disaster preparedness would be most helpful (79%) to their school to increase the emphasis on disaster preparedness. Other curriculum resources that the respondents felt would be beneficial were a competency list (55%), online course(s) (49%), train the trainers (45%), and guest speakers (40%).

These survey results validated the general assumption that nursing programs provide limited curriculum content in disaster preparedness. Also noteworthy is that most respondents felt those nursing faculties were not adequately prepared to deliver this type of content.

THE AMERICAN ORGANIZATION OF NURSE EXECUTIVES' SURVEY

The American Organization of Nurse Executives (AONE) sent a survey to its affiliated local groups to determine if a nurse leader had been made a member of the disaster management team, their background and skill acquisition, and short-comings of educational programs. As described in an e-mail (November 2002) from Jo Ann Web, RN, MHA, from AONE, 20 of 48 groups responded to the survey. The results...or capitalize on those skills. INCMCE members also developed competencies for all nurses. These competencies were developed by another task force with review and revision by INCMCE members. Current competencies can be viewed on the INCMCE website (www.incmce.org).

THE NATIONAL HEALTH PROFESSIONS PREPAREDNESS CONSORTIUM

After the establishment of INCMCE, Captain Stephens again approached the leadership of Vanderbilt University School of Nursing to join efforts with two other institutions that had an interest in educating health professionals on emergency preparedness. Vanderbilt joined with the University of Alabama Birmingham (focusing on physician education), and Louisiana State University (focusing on the emergency medical technicians [EMTs]) to merge the nursing curriculum needs. This group became the National Health Professions Preparedness Consortium (NHPPC).

The DHHS wanted a plan developed by leading institutions of higher learning involved in educating and training the nation's health professions. Consequently, NHPPC, through Auburn University, developed a 5-year strategic plan. The plan addressed the awareness, performance, and refresher needs as directed by the ACEP report [4]. Initial target audiences included nurses, physicians, and EMTs. The strategic plan's goals are:

- To provide direction for the development of the Noble Training Center, Anniston, Alabama, into a world-class academy for the training of the nation's health care providers in effective response to mass casualty incidents
- To provide direction and recommendations for developing national curricula and addressing the response preparedness of the nation's health care providers to WMD incidents and mass casualties
- To provide a process to enable DHHS, through the National Training Academy, to effectively respond and adapt to changes in threats, resources, and response strategies of the nation's health and medical communities' preparedness to respond to incidents involving WMD and mass casualties

The first course designed to achieve the goals of the plan was "Health Care and Leadership Administrative Decision-Making in Response to WMD Incidents." Students included emergency physicians and nurses, emergency medical services administrators, hospital executives, nurse executives, and nurse managers. Ongoing evaluation activities assisted the participating faculty in revising the course throughout the year. In addition, a Web-based server using BlackBoard served as the resource and communication repository for faculty and participating students throughout the year. Evaluation data before and after the NHPPC courses were gathered to determine participants' confidence to perform specific tasks related to disaster preparedness and response. Twenty-one performance standards focusing on recognition, communication, effective decision-making, integration and management of resources, and response/recovery roles during WMD incidents were evaluated [5]. Between March and August 2003, eight courses were held at the Department of Homeland Security's Noble Training Center. Paired pre- and postcourse responses were obtained from 82% of the 414 participants, who rated their ability to perform on a five-point scale ranging from 1 for poor to 5 for excellent. SAS 8.0 and SPSS 11.5 were used for data analyses. Mean pre- and post-ratings were calculated for each item and compared across courses. Difference scores between pre- and postratings were analyzed with Sign tests. The α level was set at 0.005 to control the overall type I error rate. Mean precourse statement ratings (range 1.99 to 2.91), indicated a less than adequate performance ability, whereas postcourse ratings (range 3.32 to 4.13), indicated a greater than adequate ability. All postcourse ratings were significantly higher than the precourse ratings (all $P < .001$). Variability in participant ratings between courses was assessed, and no significant difference was found for 16 of the 21 performance competencies. Results suggest a substantial improvement in perceived performance competency by participants upon completion of the course.

National Health Professions Preparedness Consortium members are developing performance level curricula for nurses, physicians, and EMTs, again with funding from DHHS. The Vanderbilt University School of Nursing is responsible for the nursing content. This project will result in development of curricula for educating nurses according to the performance level competencies designed by the INCMCE, which can be found at www.incmce.org.

Unfortunately, the establishment of the Department of Homeland Security in 2003 has created confusion as to the appropriate place for education for health care professionals in emergency preparedness and response. Other first responders fall under the jurisdiction of the Department of Homeland Security, but DHHS continues to have the mandate to educate health care professionals. As a result, the strategic 5-year plan has taken the place of many other strategic plans, on the shelf as an unfunded mandate. It is unclear how the curricular plans developed for DHHS will be updated or maintained.

IMPLICATIONS FOR ONLINE DEVELOPMENT

The most scaleable curriculum solution is one that is presented in an online Web-based format. If properly delivered, online education can be more efficient, effective, and delivered during times that are convenient for students and faculty. As a result, web based modules are being developed to reflect the INCMCE competencies.

NATIONAL CURRICULUM DEVELOPMENT EFFORTS

Two national curricular efforts will help to contribute to a critical mass of content for health care providers in emergency preparedness and response. The first is sponsored by DHHS's Health Resources and Services Administration (HRSA) and is aimed to stimulate emergency preparedness and response materials delivered in the continuing education format and as part of a health care professional curriculum. Thirty-two recipients were granted awards in September 2003. These bioterrorism training and curriculum development grants can be found on the HRSA Web site [6].

The second agency promoting educational research and development is the Agency for Health care Research and Quality (AHRQ). Its initiative was announced on May 30, 2004, and will continue annually through 2007 [7]. AHRQ intends to support research that emphasizes the following research objectives:

- Emergency preparedness of hospitals and health care systems for bioterrorism and other public health emergencies
- Enhanced capacity needs of ambulatory care, home and long-term care, care of psycho–social consequences, and other related services during and after a bioterror event and other public health emergencies
- Information technology linkages and emerging communication networks to improve the linkages between the personal health care system, emergency response networks, and public health agencies

• Novel uses of health care system training strategies that can prepare community clinicians to recognize and manage a bioterrorist event and other public health emergencies

USING "HOW PEOPLE LEARN"

A unique aspect of their development is the use of a national framework called "How People Learn" (HPL). This learning model was developed by Bransford and colleagues after a review of the educational literature [8]. The project was sponsored by the National Research Council. Bransford was a professor at Vanderbilt University and collaborated with other Vanderbilt faculty to develop interactive learning materials using this format for other projects. The application of learning science principles to mass casualty education should provide new insights into learning processes involved in workplace (rather than primarily course-based) learning, team rather than only individual learning, and performance arenas that require overwhelming success and often take place under high stress. In addition, the rapid changes in knowledge, skills, and attitudes needed for mass casualty education provide requirements for the design of environments that support much more rapid change than has been true in the past.

EVALUATION OF OUTCOMES

The Johns Hopkins University Evidence-based Practice Center was invited by the AHRQ in 2001 to summarize existing evidence on the effectiveness of training clinicians for public health events relevant to bioterrorism preparedness [9]. Clinicians were defined as all clinical health care professions, including physicians, physician assistants, nurse practitioners, nurses, and community health workers. Fig. 2 illustrates the causal pathway for bioterrorism preparedness with key questions on training clinicians [9].

The literature and Web site search identified over 1900 articles, although only 60 were found that described and evaluated an education intervention involving one of the key questions for the project. Most identified studies pertained to training clinicians for detection and management of an infectious disease outbreak. The TOPOFF (Top Officials) exercise involved a hypothetical release of plague in Denver, and was designed to test the medical and public health infrastructure in the event of an attack. Whereas this educational study was criticized for not having any specific measurable outcomes and no control group, it was the only article identified in the literature search that directly addressed and evaluated a training program in bioterrorism response. Five articles described and evaluated educational interventions pertaining to the use of hospital disaster plans. The literature suggested that disaster drill training improved knowledge of the disaster plan and allowed identification of problems in plan execution that then may be addressed. One article described a computer simulation in disaster drill training and concluded that simulation can replace expensive large-scale drills and allow identification of deficiencies in staffing, equipment, and medications. Only one study evaluated methods for

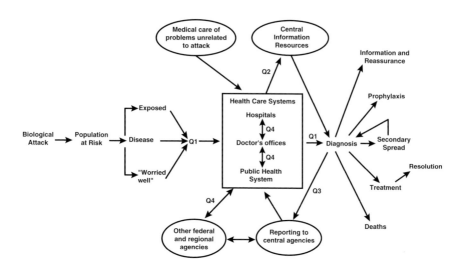

Question 1: What are effective methods for the training of clinicians for detection and management of a bioterrorist attack?

Question 2: What are effective methods for training clinicians to use web or telephone based central information resources in the event of a bioterrorist attack?

Question 3: What are effective methods for training clinicians to report events to a central agency in the event of a bioterrorist attack?

Question 4: What are effective methods for training clinicians to communicate with other health care professionals in the event of a bioterrorist attack?

Fig. 2. Causal pathway for bioterrorism preparedness with key questions on training of clinicians.

training clinicians to report events to a central agency. Educational interventions generally were more effective when they combined techniques, including interactive methods such as case discussion, simulated patients, hands-on workshops, and didactic methods.

Gaps in the literature

Three of the key questions of the study went unanswered. No literature was found that addressed the updating and reinforcing of clinician training. No literature was found that addressed the training of clinicians to use Web- or telephone-based central information sources. No literature was found on the topic of training clinicians to communicate with other health care professionals during a public health event. The authors concluded that there is a need for future research into the most effective way to train clinicians in areas that will improve their ability to respond to a bioterrorist attack or other public health event.

The Vanderbilt team led by Weiner is developing four online modules with funding from HRSA and AHRQ. The AHRQ grant focuses on the evaluation component, determining the effectiveness and efficiency of learning programs designed to educate nurses volunteering for service in their local community Medical Reserve Corps (MRC). Two types of learning programs will be compared: a face-to-face version and an online version, both of which will be designed using the principles of the national HPL framework. Effectiveness of the learning programs will be determined by: mastering course content, INCMCE competencies, incorporating principles of the HPL framework, promoting course completion, and increasing clinical confidence. Efficiency will be measured by cost per student, time spent in completion, and convenience for student. Additional aims of the project will be to define user characteristics that predict selection of and effective/efficient completion of learning programs, and to determine the adequacy of technology integration in learning emergency response content.

SUMMARY

In summary, a national model for curriculum in emergency planning and response has emerged from the work of INCMCE. Whereas several nursing programs are implementing various aspects of the competencies, there is a concerted effort to develop online modules that comprehensively address all competencies. This development is in response to a national survey of nursing programs that validated the curricular void in the area of emergency planning and response. The survey also validated that faculty development activities are needed to prepare US nursing faculty to effectively teach emergency response content. When emergency response content is compared with the INCMCE competency map, nursing organizations and individuals will be able to compare their learning needs against national nursing standards.

Implementing curricular change is not an easy task, complicated by competition for the limited time students spend in learning activities. Nursing faculty should be prepared to lead others in the emergency preparedness agenda. The increase in terrorism incidents, coupled with an increase in other natural emergencies, will be complicated further by the nursing shortage and shortage of nursing faculty. Clearly, emergency preparedness and response will continue to be an important topic for the nursing curriculum.

References

[1] American College of Emergency Physicians–NBC Task Force. Developing objectives, content, and competencies for the training of emergency medical technicians, emergency physicians, and emergency nurses to care for causalities from nuclear, biological or chemical (NBC) incidents: final report. Available at: http://www.acep.org/library/pdf/NBCreport2.pdf. Accessed April 4, 2004.

[2] Center for Health Policy. Columbia University School of Nursing. Emergency response: core competencies for all public health workers. Available at: http://www.nursing.hs.columbia.edu/institute-centers/chphsr/ERMain.html. Accessed April 4, 2004.

[3] Center for Health Policy. Columbia University. Bioterrorism & emergency readiness: competencies for all public health workers. Available at: http://www.nursing.hs.columbia.edu/institute-centers/chphsr/btcomps.pdf. Accessed April 4, 2004.

[4] National Health Professions Preparedness Consortium. Five-year strategic plan for the Noble Training Center of the United States Department of Health and Human Services; July 29, 2002. Baton Rouge (LA), NHPPC (Pursuant to Agreement with Auburn University Sub-Agreement 02-OVPR-423187).

[5] Pryor E, Heck E, Norman L, et al. Weapons of mass destruction (WMD) hospital leadership course: evaluation of participant response capabilities. Presented at the Harvard University BioSecurity 2003 Conference. Washington (DC), October 20–22, 2003.

[6] Health Resources and Services Administration. Bioterrorism training and curriculum development grants. Available at: (http://www.hrsa.gov/bioterrorism.htm). Accessed April 4, 2004.

[7] Agency for Healthcare Research and Quality. Building the evidence to promote bioterrorism and other public health emergency preparedness in health care systems. Available at: http://grants1.nih.gov/grants/guide/pa-files/PAR-03-130.html. Accessed April 4, 2004.

[8] National Research Council. How people learn: brain, mind, experience, and school. Committee on Developments in the Science of Learning. In: Bransford JD, Brown AL, Cocking RR, editors. Commission of Behavioral and Social Sciences and Education. Washington (DC): National Academy Press; 2000. p. 131–54.

[9] Johns Hopkins Evidence-based Practice Center. Training of clinicians for public health events relevant to bioterrorism preparedness; 2002. Rockville (MD), Agency for Healthcare Research and Quality, AHRQ Publication #02-E011.

[10] University of Ulster. School of Health Sciences, Nursing. Course document for postgraduate diploma/MSc in disaster relief nursing for entry. Ulster (UK): 1999. Available at: http://prospectus.ulster.ac.uk/course/?id=2137.

Nurs Clin N Am 40 (2005) 481–497

NURSING CLINICS
OF NORTH AMERICA

ELSEVIER
SAUNDERS

Homeland Security Challenges in Nursing Practice

Connie Boatright, MSN, RN[a,b,*],
K. Joanne McGlown, RN, MHHA, CHE, PhD[c]

[a]Indiana Primary Health Care Association, 1006 E. Washington Street, Suite 200,
Indianapolis, IN 46202, USA
[b]National AMEDD Augmentation Detachment, US Army Reserve, 1401 Deschler Street SW,
Fort McPherson, GA 30330, USA
[c]University of Alabama at Birmingham, Birmingham, AL, USA

At the same time as the nation's health care industry prepares for the new environment of homeland security challenges, the nursing profession also must learn and adapt. Nursing must integrate information and processes into an already challenged climate if it is to maintain credibility and emerge as a leader. Existing clinical knowledge possessed by most nurses forms an adequate baseline for building skills required to practice in the new environment, and nurses indeed are actively involved in emerging training opportunities. Nurses are less engaged, however, in critical activities related to legislation, policy, systems, and regulations that drive and sustain practice and that are essential to mastering challenges of the new environment.

The greatest volume of policy-level activity surrounding health care's role in homeland security seems to be occurring at the state level or higher. By far the largest health care professional group, nursing is under-represented where national legislation is defended and passed, state and community programs are determined, and critical regulatory and policy decisions are made that influence practice. Perhaps as great a challenge to nursing as preparing for homeland security issues is that of expanding its role and elevating its level of influence well beyond the clinical care arena. Nurses need a comprehensive knowledge of doctrine, laws, regulations, programs, and processes that build the operational framework for health care preparedness. Key components of this knowledge base reside in the areas of evolution of homeland security—laws and mandates affecting health care and compliance—and regulatory issues for health care organizations.

*Corresponding author: 5301 Lancelot Drive Indianapolis, Indiana 46228, USA.
E-mail address: cboatright@ori.net (C. Boatright).

0029-6465/05/$ – see front matter
doi:10.1016/j.cnur.2005.04.003

This article addresses primary components in both of these areas, after first assessing the status of nursing's involvement (in homeland security), as portrayed in the professional literature.

NURSING'S CONTRIBUTIONS TO HOMELAND SECURITY AS DEPICTED IN THE LITERATURE

A useful gauge of assessing where any professional group's involvement and power reside at any point in time is the prevalence of that group's representation in the professional literature. A simple database assessment indicated that nursing content in the areas of terrorism and bioterrorism are almost nonexistent.

The scientific literature is rife with accounts of the health care industry's attempt to determine how best to integrate new requirements and demands in an already challenged environment. The level of nursing's activity is not yet apparent in the respected academic and peer-reviewed journals. A recent review of the literature revealed that no one academic or trade journal, in either the nursing or health administration fields, has emerged as a source for current and frequent information relevant to planning and preparedness for emergency or disaster situations, at least not on the topic of bioterrorism.

A February 2004, literature search using two primary health care and nursing literature databases, OVID [1] and CINAHL [2], searched the keyword bioterrorism and articles published in English. The findings were unexpected and disheartening for the nursing profession. Searching OVID for articles published in English from October 2001, to February 2004, revealed over 1200 different items. A subjective selection of articles appearing most focused on terrorism or disaster preparedness resulted in 148 articles from 30 distinct health-related journals. The articles fell into nine different categories. The largest percentage of articles was on general aspects of bioterrorism (37.2%), public health law, ethics and policy issues (14.8%), and preparedness (12.2%). Nursing's role in a bioterrorism response was covered in only 17 articles (11.5%) of the total. The greatest number of articles per journal appeared in two instances. Seven articles each were identified from a special issue of *Emergency Medicine Clinics of North America*, and from the *American Journal of Nursing*. Four other periodicals followed with five articles each. Forty-nine (N = 49) journals published only one article on the subject in the 2.5 years since the events of Sept. 11, 2001.

An identical search in the CINAHL database for nursing and allied health literature revealed 157 articles of significance. Most (73 articles, 47%) were general bioterrorism articles, while 13.4% (N = 21) discussed public health or health care law, policy issues, and the federal government. The nursing-specific articles on the topic were very similar to the OVID search, with 10.8% of the total devoted to nursing aspects. No one journal emerged as a prominent source for articles on the topics of planning and preparedness for current threats. The 17 articles the authors found of greatest interest came from 13 different journals, with the greatest number of citations per journal at three. Fourteen of the total 17 journals (82%) published only one article each.

Although not an exhaustive search, this account illustrates the absence of nursing involvement, or nursing's portrayal of its involvement, in published forums read by practicing nurses and others affected by the health care industry's war on terrorism. Nurse leaders and academicians need to conduct credible research and encourage and support others to contribute to the literature. In addition to gaining professional credibility and visibility through the sharing of ideas, programs, and practice issues, nursing will benefit from the enhanced visibility of the profession through external recognition and inclusion as subject matter experts in arenas where decisions are made and resources allocated.

KEY KNOWLEDGE BASE AREAS

Two areas of importance for nursing to expand its knowledge and influence in homeland security are those pertaining to the evolution of homeland security laws and mandates impacting health care, and compliance and regulatory issues for health care organizations.

Evolution of homeland security: laws and mandates impacting health care

Long before America's leaders developed national plans, enacted legislation, and formed departments and agencies to address the impact of terrorism, they recognized that the country was ill-prepared to manage consequences of catastrophic events of any cause. Although the United States has yet to experience a natural disaster or other nonterrorist event resulting in massive numbers of casualties of the magnitude experienced in foreign countries, it has had close calls and longitudinally has tallied significant casualty counts. From 1975 to 1994, natural hazards (eg, earthquakes, hurricanes, floods, and tornadoes) in the United States and its territories resulted in more than 24,000 deaths and approximately 100,000 injuries. (Since that tally, deaths and injuries resulting from natural hazards have occurred, although not in numbers that overwhelmed the country's response resources.) The trend of increases in disaster losses is expected to continue [3], and numbers of people affected by disasters will continue to increase. This trend has prompted the US Government to further develop and refine its nationwide preparedness strategy.

Several key initiatives have evolved that direct how the United States and its health care systems manage those affected by disaster and catastrophic events. These include the National Disaster Medical System (NDMS), National Response Plan (NRP), Robert T. Stafford Disaster Relief and Emergency Assistance Act, Strategic National Stockpile, Metropolitan Medical Response System (MMRS), Weapons of Mass Destruction (WMD) Act of 1996, Homeland Security Act of 2004, various homeland security presidential directives (HSPDs) and bioterrorism funding initiatives.

National Disaster Medical System

One of the most robust national initiatives with significance to the health care industry is the NDMS. In 1984, the Reagan administration recognized the lack of an organized approach to managing mass casualties resulting from disaster or other catastrophic event. This realization resulted in the formation of NDMS. A massive partnership among federal agencies, the initial NDMS partners included the Department of Health and Human Services (DHHS)/US Public Health Service (PHS), Department of Veterans Affairs (VA), Department of Defense (DoD) and Federal Emergency Management Agency (FEMA) [4]. The recent realignment of FEMA under the newly formed Department of Homeland Security (DHS) has resulted in DHS replacing FEMA as an NDMS partner. NDMS first was recognized in public law in the PHS and Bioterrorism Preparedness and Response Act (PL 107-188) of 2002 [5].

The National Disaster Medical System groups patients into five categories, compatible with classifications used by DoD, when providing medical evacuation of casualties of war or catastrophic events. These are: medical–surgical, critical care, pediatric, burn, and psychiatric [6]. The three missions of NDMS are: field medical response, patient transport, and definitive care [4].

National disaster medical system field medical response. National disaster medical system field medical response is provided by disaster medical assistance teams (DMATs) comprised of clinical and support volunteers who train for and agree to deploy during disaster response and recovery activities. These volunteer teams consist of nurses, doctors, and allied health and support personnel from throughout the country who become federalized when deployed in an NDMS activation. Deployed staffs are paid and receive legal coverage for personal practice liability under the Federal Tort Claims Act, and are reimbursed for travel, lodging, and meal expenses. DMAT members receive extensive training for the roles they will fill. Deployments generally involve being absent from the member's primary duty or employment site for 14 days.

Two other types of NDMS teams have been deployed following disasters or terrorist events. Disaster mortuary teams (DMORTs), comprised of funeral directors, forensics specialists, pathologists, and other supporting members, provide body recovery services and identification and security of remains at the disaster site. Veterinary assistance teams (VMATs), comprised of veterinarians and related personnel, provide care for rescue animals in disasters.

Patient transport. Patient transport manages the flow of patients to ensure the appropriate distribution of casualties and provides transport and tracking of victims from the disaster area to lesser-impacted areas. DoD is responsible for patient transport in a federally declared disaster. Long-distance transport usually is provided by US Air Force aircraft but also can be accomplished by commercial air, rail, bus, or other means. The transport component is formalized through memoranda of understanding (MOUs) between NDMS representatives with airports, local emergency medical services (EMS), and civilian hospitals that ultimately receive and treat referred casualties.

Definitive care. The third NDMS component, definitive care, expands the public and private hospital bed capacity by identifying civilian/community hospitals that agree to provide staffed beds for victims of disaster or other catastrophic events. Approximately 1800 United States health care facilities have formal MOUs with NDMS for this purpose and are referred to as NDMS-enrolled facilities. Most larger, comprehensive hospitals or medical centers in the United States are enrolled in NDMS. MOUs define how facilities will receive victims and be reimbursed for services.

Federal coordinating centers (FCCs) provide oversight and coordination of NDMS bed availability, and are located at VA medical centers (VAMCs) or DoD medical centers in 70 locations throughout the country. VA and DoD FCC representatives conduct routinely scheduled bed counts, where civilian NDMS-enrolled health care facilities report available staffed beds in the five specialty categories to DoD. Consistent bed reporting exercises are critical for planning, as available staffed bed numbers may fluctuate depending on local demands (eg, influenza epidemics and other diseases) that may result in critical bed shortages in areas of the country [4].

Individual elements of NDMS have been activated, but the DHHS assistant secretary of health never has activated the entire system fully for domestic emergencies. DMATs, DMORTs, and other NDMS field medical response components have mobilized many times in support of disasters declared by the president, mass casualty or fatality incidents, and high-visibility national security events (eg, economic summits, large sporting events, and presidential inaugurations). Following the Sept. 11, 2001, terrorist attacks, although some DMAT assets were deployed, the numbers of live victims requiring care did not exceed local resource capabilities. DMORTs were deployed and were the federal groups most engaged in the 9/11 response and recovery.

National Response Plan

The National Response Plan (NRP) (originally termed The Federal Response Plan) was a new document in 1992 when Hurricane Andrew devastated Miami-Dade County, Florida. The hundreds of responders and providers who first applied the plan during that event validated its utility as an effective guide for an overwhelming natural disaster event. The NRP is FEMA's formal approach to managing disaster response and recovery, addressing several needs and services.

The original plan, focusing on natural disasters, assigned responsibility for 12 categories of support to 28 different federal agencies, with FEMA serving as the lead federal agency (LFA) [7]. The NRP now includes 15 categories, or emergency support functions (ESFs), and each cites an LFA and supporting agencies. Over 30 federal agencies and the American Red Cross (ARC) now support the FRP [8]. The 15 ESFs address specific areas, allowing the agencies assigned to each ESF to focus specifically on the single ESF mission. Before the NRP (FRP), there were often difficulties with resource allocation and confusion over which agency was in charge of specific tasks.

Of most relevance and interest to health care and nursing is "ESF #8: Public Health and Medical Services," with DHHS serving as LFA supported by a host of other agencies. ESF #8 addresses many functions that involve morbidity and mortality associated with disaster or other catastrophic events. On-scene medical response, epidemiological issues, water, food and vector control, and numerous health and medical needs are addressed by ESF #8 activation. Another ESF of interest to health care providers and nursing is ESF #6: Mass Care, Housing and Human Services, led by the ARC, the only nonfederal agency with a Congressional mandated role in disaster response and the only one to lead an ESF. ESF #6 is activated in situations where large numbers of victims require temporary shelter, feeding and mental health and related services. The ARC can mobilize a nationwide cadre of volunteer licensed nurses, mental health counselors, and other health specialists to perform these missions.

The NRP also includes a series of annexes to address incident-specific guidelines. In 1998, a terrorism annex was added to the FRP [5]. With the formation of DHS (and its oversight of FEMA), the NRP has been revised to reflect these organizational changes and additional annexes.

The Stafford Act

The Robert T. Stafford Disaster Relief and Emergency Assistance Act (PL100-107), as amended, provides federal assistance to states for managing the consequences of disasters by expediting the rendering of aid, assistance, and emergency services, and the reconstruction and rehabilitation of devastated areas. Although the Stafford Act does not provide direct funding for health and medical issues, reimbursement for expenditures may be possible following specific guidelines.

Strategic national stockpile

Managed by the Centers for Disease Control and Prevention (CDC) with the support of VA, the Strategic National Stockpile (SNS) provides life-saving pharmaceuticals, antidotes, and other medical supplies and equipment for use in a biological terrorist event within the country. Whereas the SNS is specific to biological agent exposure, there also exists strategically located pharmaceutical stockpiles for use by DHHS national medical response teams (NMRTs), designed to treat victims of chemical and other terrorist attacks. The stationery locations of these stockpiles are classified [9], although the contents can be relocated quickly proximal to a high-risk area or actual terrorist event. Many VAMCs throughout the country also have pharmaceutical caches, intended for use with veteran patients; however, these caches could be requested in response to a community-wide incident where life and health could be compromised. Having knowledge of stockpile or cache existence is an important component to nursing knowledge. Nurses could be called upon to assist with activation and preparation of a stockpile, organize and work within a predesigned drug delivery administration system in their community, and administer agents.

The Metropolitan Medical Response System

Where the NDMS is considered a top-down approach to disaster response, the metropolitan medical response system MMRS is a bottom-up approach.

Established in 1996, the MMRS was developed to enhance local emergency preparedness systems for response to a public health crisis, particularly one involving weapons of mass destruction (WMD), until federal resources arrive (typically 24 to 48 hours). By late 2002, DHHS had funded 122 local jurisdictions to facilitate the preparation and coordination of public health, medical and mental health, local law enforcement, emergency management, and first responders to more effectively respond in the first 48 to 72 hours of a public health crisis.

The Metropolitan Medical Response System has directly supported the linkages among local elements essential to managing a WMD mass casualty event. MMRS coordinates or is involved in initiatives in major metropolitan areas for chemical, biological, or nuclear agent identification; medical intelligence gathering and distribution; patient triage and treatment capability and support; mass prophylaxis of affected populations; mass fatality management; enhanced emergency transport capabilities; integration with federal resources (NDMS, SNS); patient decontamination capability and support; and coordination of patient transportation to receiving facilities. MMRS performs all operations through local professional volunteers. Although the MMRS focus is on terrorist events, MMRS assets also can enhance local capabilities in the event of hazardous materials (HAZMAT) incidents, natural disaster, and disease outbreaks [10].

Since the formation of DHS, national coordination and management of MMRS funding and guidance, like many federal programs, has undergone changes in alignment and in how grants are administered. In 2004, the MMRS program was folded under the Office of State and Local Government Coordination and Preparedness, Office for Domestic Preparedness, in keeping with the DHS goal of establishing a more streamlined administration system for state, local, and tribal nation grants. MMRS programs and grant guidance and funding are coordinated by the State Administration Agency in each State [11].

Weapons of Mass Destruction Act of 1996
Many believe that the attacks of Sept. 11, 2001, were the defining wake-up call for United States preparedness for terrorism, but efforts had begun long before 2002. Senators Nunn, Lugar, and Domenici, concerned with the growing instability of rogue nations and their access to WMD, acted to increase efforts for United States preparedness. The 1995 sarin nerve agent attack on the Tokyo subway system and attempt in the early 1990s to destroy the World Trade Towers in New York City further emphasized the importance of terrorism preparedness in the United States. The 1996 Defense Authorization Act provided funding for equipment and training for local first responders for the effective management of incidents involving WMD through the Domestic Preparedness Program. DoD developed and delivered the Domestic Preparedness Program in the nation's largest 120 largest cities, followed by training in smaller communities for first responders and health care facility staff [5].

The Homeland Security Act of 2002 (Public Law 107-296)
This act, signed into law November 2002, created the DHS, consolidating many functions of various departments and agencies under a single department. It is considered the largest federal government reorganization in over a 50 years [5].

Homeland Security presidential directives
Each president issues presidential directives under his watch. In February 2003, President George W. Bush signed Homeland Security Presidential Directive (HSPD) #5, which directs the development of a national incident management system; establishes a unified command system for national response; and renames the Federal Response Plan to the National Response Plan [5].

The relevance of HSPD #5 to health care and nursing is in the manner in which responses will be managed. As health care facilities and systems become more engaged in the management of a consolidated response, they may be required to learn new ways of functioning in a crisis.

Also of importance to health care organizations are HSPD #8 and #9 [5]. HSPD #8, published Dec. 17, 2003, describes the way federal departments and agencies will prepare for a response, including prevention during early stages of a terrorist event. The DHS secretary will coordinate implementation of all-hazards preparedness, coordinate preparedness of federal response assets, and support an assessment of the preparedness of state and local first responders. HSPD #8 mandates the development of a national domestic all-hazards preparedness goal by 2006. This goal will provide measurable readiness priorities and targets that balance threats with resources, and will include metrics for readiness. For the first time, measurable all-hazards preparedness goals will be mandated nationally. For state and local providers to meet these goals, all responder agencies, including the health care and medical sectors, must participate in such planning actively.

Homeland Security presidential directive number 9, new for 2004, included hospitals as first responders, along with the traditional agencies such as EMS, fire, and law enforcement. This may prove essential for health care organizations, as hospitals now may be allowed to apply for government grants for training and education, monies that have been denied the health care industry to this point. With expanded requirements for internal drills and training (eg, Joint Commission on Accreditation of Healthcare Organization [JCAHO] standards) and expectations of external participation in exercises, the health care industry has been hard-hit by these unfunded mandates and will benefit from the opportunity to seek funding assistance as they strive to address current and future needs.

Bioterrorism funding
Since Sept. 11, 2001, the federal government has instituted critical programs that focus on health care planning and preparedness for incidents involving bioterrorism and other mass casualties.

HEALTH RESOURCES AND SERVICES ADMINISTRATION NATIONAL BIOTERRORISM HOSPITAL PREPAREDNESS PROGRAM

In 2002, DHHS's Health Resources and Services Administration began providing funding to public health departments for the development of programs to prepare hospitals and related entities for response to bioterrorism and non-terrorist events involving infectious disease and epidemics. The focus is on bioterrorism preparedness plans and protocols for hospitals and other health care entities [12]. The primary purpose of the grant awards is development and implementation of regional plans that enhance capacity of hospitals, emergency departments, community health centers, outpatient centers, EMS systems, rural health clinics, and other health care systems and programs for response to incidents where mass immunization, treatment, quarantine, isolation, and other measures may be essential following a bioterrorism or infectious disease event.

COOPERATIVE AGREEMENT ON PUBLIC HEALTH PREPAREDNESS AND RESPONSE FOR BIOTERRORISM

The CDC's cooperative agreement focuses on public health preparedness and response for bioterrorism, but it includes many components that extend beyond public health and into the larger health care community. The grant program's intent is to upgrade preparedness and response of local and state public health jurisdictions in their potential roles with bioterrorism and other infectious disease outbreaks or public health emergencies [13]. Each state receiving funds is required to both develop a statewide plan outlining how it will respond to a bioterrorism or infectious disease incident and on how it will enhance core public health capacities. The program cites several areas for improvement: planning and readiness assessment; surveillance and epidemiology; laboratory capacity-biologic agents; healthalert network/communications and information technology; communicating health risks and health information dissemination; and education and training.

Program funding is provided through state public health departments to local communities, where regional or local coordinators have responsibility to work with health care entities in improving capability in the aforementioned areas.

These federally (HRSA/CDC) funded grant programs have been instrumental in building programs and relationships in local and state health care arenas, resulting in close collaboration among various health care entities and between health care and other emergency management entities.

COMPLIANCE AND REGULATORY ISSUES FOR HEALTH CARE ORGANIZATIONS

Emergency management, safety, and security activities in hospitals and other health care facilities are subject to oversight and guidance from several federal regulating agencies. These become even more critical when addressing issues of preparedness and response to potential terrorist events. Standards and guidelines from the Occupational Safety and Health Administration (OSHA), Environmental Protection Agency (EPA) and the National Fire Protection Association (NFPA) or many of the federal acts and laws that govern response in hazardous environments may not be familiar to most nursing professionals. Their strength in guiding the behavior of health care organizations, however, cannot be ignored.

The enhancement and strengthening of all-hazards emergency and disaster planning and preparedness in America's health care facilities was, in most cases, encouraged by the desire to meet accreditation standards of JCAHO or the public health guidelines of each state. Nurses in all specialties and roles need a working knowledge of these expectations to enhance understanding and facilitate preparedness for disasters, whether natural or man-made.

Joint Commission on Accreditation of Healthcare Organizations

In its 2004 survey guidelines for health care facilities (but excluding behavioral health), JCAHO provided five primary expectations over seven risk categories [14]. The seven environment of care (EC) risk categories are: general safety, security, hazardous materials and waste, emergency management, fire safety, medical/laboratory equipment, and utilities. The expectations of organizations within these categories are reflected in Box 1. Although emergency management requirements are stated in several places, the primary standards are found in EC.1.0 through EC.9.30.

In 2000, JCAHO required that health care organization plans address comprehensive emergency management (CEM), the four phases of which describe the emergency management cycle in the United States. Although some feel the standards are self-explanatory, the 2004 version clearly illustrates that the rationale and elements of performance for each standard must be

---

Box 1: Joint Commission on Accreditation of Healthcare Organizations expectations of organization in the seven risk categories

Conduct a hazard vulnerability analysis.

Identify your role in relation to the community's, county's, or region's emergency management program.

Identify processes to ensure that information is shared in a timely manner from hospitals and long-term care facilities with other health care organizations that provide services within the contiguous geographic area.

Identify an all-hazards command structure that links with that of the community.

Make needed improvements and alterations in emergency plans based on critiques of emergency management drills and exercises.

From Joint Commission on Accreditation of Healthcare Organizations (JCAHO). Environment of Care News 2003;6(12).

considered and addressed to ensure compliance. With very few exceptions, all aspects of the standards are relevant to ensuring preparedness of a safe, all-hazards environment, designed to enhance nursing function and protect patient care in and following disasters and situations of risk. Table 1 illustrates the CEM phases and program elements under each phase.

Although found primarily in the EC standards, relevant standards for disaster preparedness are also found in the leadership (LD), surveillance, prevention and control of infection (IC) standards, human resources (HR), and medical staff (MS) standards, among others. Table 2 summarizes the JCAHO standards most relevant to emergency management and disaster preparedness.

The Joint Commission on Accreditation of Healthcare Organizations requires nurse managers and other executives of the health care facility to possess a broad knowledge of specific expectations for preparedness and response for all-hazards disasters. Among the most critical is the performance of a risk and hazards vulnerability assessment on which to base further planning. New approaches emerge with regularity, requiring quick research and study to improve knowledge and the ability to develop and implement the most current practices. Some of these include knowledge of personal protective equipment (PPE), shelter-in-place and evacuation procedures, mass vaccination

Table 1	
Comprehensive emergency management	

CEM Phases

CEM has been a cornerstone of the Federal Emergency Management Agency (FEMA) program policy since the agency's creation in 1979. CEM integrates various emergency programs and activities into a life cycle. The four phases are visualized as a circle, with one phase leading to the next, and allowing phases to overlap when required.

Phase	Program elements
Mitigation	Hazards identification and risk assessment
	Hazards management
	Public education and information
Preparedness	Resource management
	Planning
	Training
	Exercises, evaluation, and corrective action
	Finance and administration
Response	Direction, control, and coordination
	Communications and warning
	Operations and procedures
	Logistics and facilities
Recovery	Short- and long-term priorities and procedures
	Vital resources
	Resumption/restoration procedures

Data from Brewster P. NFPA 1600 elements aligned with CEM phases. Indianapolis (IN): Emergency Management Strategic Healthcare Group, Department of Veterans Affairs, 2001.

Table 2
Select Joint Commission on Accreditation of Healthcare Organizations 2004 standards relevant to disaster planning and preparedness

Standard	Statement	Includes
EC.1.10	Hospital manages safety risks	Safe environment Safety planning, implementation, and worker safety
EC.1.20	Safe environment	Is maintained
EC.1.30	Hospital develops and implements prohibition of smoking	No smoking policies implemented, monitored with proven corrective action taken
EC.2.10	Identifies and manages security risks	Plans and implements a secure environment
EC.3.10	Manages hazardous materials and waste risks	
EC.4.10	Addresses emergency management	Planning and implementation of an emergency management plan
EC.4.20	Drills regularly to test emergency management	
EC.5.10 EC.5.40 EC.5.50	Fire safety risks, maintains equipment and building safety	Development of a risk management plan, takes action to protect occupants
EC.5.20 EC.5.30	Compliance with life safety codes Fire drills conducted regularly	
EC.6.10 EC.6.20	Medical equipment	Risks addressed, equipment maintained and inspected
EC.7.10 EC.7.20 EC.7.30 EC.7.40 EC.7.50	Utility risks Reliable emergency electrical power source; utility, medical gas, vacuum, and emergency power systems	Risks addressed, systems maintained and inspected
EC.8.10 EC.8.30	Appropriate environment, even through renovation or construction	Establishes and maintains
EC.9.10 EC.9.20 EC.9.30	Monitors overall safety environment, identifies and addresses issues of concern for improvement	Reporting, monitoring, annual evaluations, and improvement to a safe environment
HR.2.13	Patient security, confidentiality, and privacy	Establishes and maintains
HR2.20	Personnel know their roles and responsibilities relative to safety	EC education and staff knowledge requirements
RI.1.10	Ethical behavior	In care, treatment, services, and business practices
MS3.10	Medical staff	Role in hospital improvement activities and patient safety
IC.1.10-6.30 IC.3.10	Surveillance, prevention, and control of infection standards	Identification, control, and risk reduction; reporting to public health agencies

Standard	Statement	Includes
Table 2 (continued)		
LD1.30 LD.1.3.4	Hospital complies with laws and regulations, serves the community	Shows commitment to community by providing essential services in timely manner
LD.3.60 LD.4.40	Effective communication system	Leaders provide facility-wide communication
LD.4.50	Leaders role in unusual or urgent events	Identify how priorities are adjusted and set performance improvement priorities, including facility-wide patient safety program

Data from Joint Commission on Accreditation of Healthcare Organizations. Crosswalks of 2003 standards to 2004 standards. 2004 Hospital accreditation standards. Oakbrook (IL): JCAHO; 2004. p. 337–83.

and inoculation, and planning based on an incident command or management system (ICS/IMS).

INCIDENT COMMAND SYSTEM/INCIDENT MANAGEMENT SYSTEM

The ICS is a systems approach to managing an emergency situation where more than one organization or entity is involved. ICS, now called IMS, was developed in the mid-1970s by the fire service and became the model for managing wild land fires involving response from multiple states, jurisdictions, and agencies. IMS has become the nationally accepted standard for managing emergencies. As cited earlier, HSPD-5 requires that applicable federal agencies adopt IMS. IMS is organized by functions, arranging all services and personnel under the distinct functional areas of planning, operations, logistics, and finance. Most responder/clinical staff align under the operations function. All functional area leaders report to the incident manager (commander). The success of IMS lies in its key provisions of:

- Common terminology
- Integrated communications
- Modular organization
- Unified management structure
- Manageable span of control
- Consolidated action plans
- Comprehensive resource management [5]

These features provide tremendous benefits for those responding, in that one is not required to be responsible for knowing all aspects of a response. Rather the responder need only be focused on her/his duties (job descriptions are provided) and know to whom to report.

Popularity of IMS/ICS has expanded to the health care facility setting, where the Hospital Emergency Incident Management System (HEICS) and similar models now are used increasingly [15]. All hospitals should be implementing IMS, HEICS, or some form of IMS that conforms to that practiced throughout the community. Although JCAHO accreditation is a frequent and powerful driver of health care organization behavior, there are many additional laws, regulations, guidelines, and standards that also must be considered in developing comprehensive disaster and response plans.

Superfund Amendments and Reauthorization Act, Title III (1986)

One of the early, yet more significant, acts to require community action to address potential threats was the Superfund Amendments and Reauthorization Act (SARA) of 1986, Title III. SARA, Title III, the Emergency Planning and Community Right-to-Know Act requires notifications to state and local agencies concerning the hazardous materials and substances present in the community. Community-wide emergency planning for the release of chemical agents is required, and the development of local response plans and procedures are facilitated through the establishment of the local emergency planning committees (LEPCs) and state emergency response commissions (SERCs). Health care organizations should be active participants in this collaborative planning effort [16].

Hazardous Waste Operations and Emergency Response

Occupational Safety and Health Administration regulations affect nurses through their key regulations for hazardous materials incidents (29CFR Part 1910). The Hazardous Waste Operations and Emergency Response (HAZW-OPER) regulation applies to hospitals in scenarios involving release of a hazardous material, as do PPE and toxic and hazardous substances regulations.

Environmental Protection Agency

Environmental Protection Agency regulations affect health care organizations and the nurses who will respond through guidelines for PPE, decontamination, and the environmental consequences of the run-off from the decontamination process. Nurses most likely will lead preparation for the receipt of contaminated patients, and their stabilization and treatment.

Other regulations

Many standards from several other agencies also address multiple and mass casualty incidents and should be considered when developing comprehensive plans for health care organizations.

American National Standards Institute

The American Standards Institute accredits the NFPA and provides standards for electrical safety, information management, and operational standards for hazardous materials incidents [17].

American Society of Testing and Materials
Standard F-1288, the Standard Guide for Planning for and Responding to a Multiple Casualty Incident (MCI), covers planning, needs assessment, training, interagency coordination, mutual aid, and other issues [18].

National Fire Protection Association
Before JCAHO's action to require emergency plan development and preparations to fully integrate health care organizations with the efforts of the community, the NFPA realized the lag and established standards for health care facilities through Standard 99, Chapter 12 (Health Care Facility Emergency Management) [19] and Standard 1600 (Emergency Management and Business Continuity Programs). Standard 1600 established the basis for the emergency management program evaluation and accreditation system in use by many state, local, and tribal governments. It represents the first and early standard for community-wide emergency management programs [20]. Although individual facilities may be accredited by JCAHO, it is still wise to review the NFPA standards to ensure compliance with these guidelines.

SUMMARY

The nursing profession has an opportunity and a responsibility to become involved in policy and legislative processes that impact homeland security programs, particularly those related to health care. The largest and most diverse group of health care professionals, nurses certainly will be involved in the response to and recovery from most terrorist or mass casualty events. By adopting a comprehensive emergency management approach, nursing can advance from its traditional roles in response and recovery to the expanded roles that include preparedness and mitigation activities. To do this, the profession must keep in step with the volume of evolving legislation on homeland security, with particular attention to laws and mandates that impact health care and how they translate to state and local programs. Additionally, nursing must become attuned to homeland security-related policy and regulatory issues for hospitals, community health centers, public health agencies, and other applicable arenas.

Familiarity with emerging laws and policies is only an initial step toward nursing establishing itself as a recognized leader in health care aspects of homeland security. Examples of initiatives and programs where nursing involvement and leadership can contribute include:

- Inclusion of homeland security courses, competencies and curricula in schools of nursing
- Rotation of undergraduate and graduate nursing students through public health, emergency management, government, and related programs involved in homeland security
- Participation in and volunteering for leadership roles in local and state forums that address homeland security as applied to health care issues (eg, HRSA state and district bioterrorism meetings)

- • Contributing to the professional literature through sharing of concepts and programs and ideas for best practices and scientific inquiry
- • Developing and delivering relevant education and training in the workplace, community, and beyond
- • Active participation on hospital- and community-based organized teams (eg, decontamination teams that focus on homeland security events)
- • In addition to mentoring and directing students and practicing nurses, established nursing academicians and leaders are positioned to provide leadership through service on applicable policy-level committees and forums focused on homeland security in health care.

All Americans are challenged with the new reality resulting from terrorism and potential future threats. One of nursing's greatest challenges is determining how best to carve the profession's direction, while significantly influencing health care's role in homeland security at all levels.

References

[1] Technologies OVID Incorporated. Available at: http://www.ovid.com. Accessed May 5, 2004.

[2] Information Systems CINAHL. Available at: http://www.cinahl.com. Accessed May 5, 2004.

[3] Mileti D. Disasters by design: a reassessment of natural hazards in the United States. Brookfield (CT): Rothstein Associates; 1999. p. 4–5.

[4] Brandt EN Jr, Mayer WN, Mason JO, et al. Designing a national disaster medical system. Public Health Rep 1985;100(5):455–61.

[5] Barbisch DM, Boatright CB. Understanding the government's role in emergency management. In: McGlown KJ, editor. Terrorism and disaster management: preparing healthcare for the new reality. Chicago: Health Administration Press; 2004. p. 149–75.

[6] Boatright CB. The rc–va connection: defending and protecting the nation's health and safety. The Officer 2003;LXXIX(9):67–9.

[7] Federal Emergency Management Agency (FEMA). Federal response plan. Washington (DC): FEMA; 1992.

[8] Department of Homeland Security. National response plan. Washington (DC): Department of Homeland Security; 2004.

[9] Veterans Health Administration. Emergency management program guidebook. Washington (DC): Department of Veterans Affairs; 2002.

[10] National Disaster Medical System. US Public Health Service. Field operations guide for metropolitan medical response team. Rockville (MD): US Public Health Service; 1998.

[11] Department of Homeland Security. Available at: http://www.mmrs.fema.gov. Accessed January 6, 2005.

[12] Health Resources and Services Administration. National bioterrorism hospital preparedness program cooperative agreement guidance. Rockville (MD): US Department of Health and Human Services; 2003.

[13] Centers for Disease Control and Prevention. Continuation guidance for cooperative agreement on public health preparedness and response for bioterrorism. Atlanta (GA): Department of Health and Human Services; 2003.

[14] Joint Commission on Accreditation of Healthcare Organizations. Environment of Care News 2003;6(12).

[15] California Emergency Medical Services Authority. Hospital emergency incident command system. Sacramento (CA): California Emergency Medical Services; 1998.

[16] Tierney KJ, Lindell MK, Perry RW. Facing the unexpected: disaster preparedness and response in the United States. Washington (DC): John Henry Press; 2001. p. 62–3.

[17] Occupational Safety and Health Administration. Occupational safety and health standards; subpart H – hazardous materials. 1910.120: hazardous waste operations and emergency response. Code of Federal Regulations, Title 2, Sec. 1910. Washington (DC): Occupational Safety and Health Administration; 2003.

[18] American Society of Testing and Materials (ASTM). Standard guide for planning for and response to multiple casualty incidents. ASTM 1288. Committee F30 on Emergency Medical Services. Washington (DC): ASTM International; 1990.

[19] National Fire Protection Association. Healthcare facility emergency management. Standard 99(12). Quincy (MA): National Fire Protection Association; 2002.

[20] National Fire Protection Association. Emergency management and business continuity programs. Standard 1600. Quincy (MA): National Fire Protection Association; 2002.

Nurs Clin N Am 40 (2005) 499–509

NURSING CLINICS
OF NORTH AMERICA

ELSEVIER
SAUNDERS

The Role of Public Health Nursing in Emergency Preparedness and Response

Rosemarie Rowney, MPH, RN[a],*, Georgia Barton, MA, RN[b]

[a]Schools of Nursing and Public Health; Bioterrorism Preparedness Initiative,
University of Michigan, 400 North Ingalls, Room 4162, Ann Arbor, MI 48109, USA
[b]University of Michigan School of Nursing, 400 North Ingalls, Room 4155, Ann Arbor,
MI 48109, USA

Public health services are considered integral to homeland security and defense, and public health workers are at the forefront of emergency preparedness and response [1]. Anthrax threats and scares and the emergence of new infectious diseases such as West Nile virus, severe acute respiratory syndrome (SARS), and avian influenza have put an increased focus on the essential functions of the country's public health infrastructure. Nurses make up the largest group of health care professionals who work in state and local public health departments across the nation [2] and provide a wide range of services. The new challenges for public health come at a time when there are fewer resources to support such efforts.

The increased need for public health services comes at a time when the current national public health infrastructure of 3000 local health departments has been weakened by years of financial and administrative neglect. There appears to be a lack of funding or political will to support population-based interventions for promoting health and preventing disease. The public health workforce is challenged to function as first responders (ie, the initial health care professionals who contact victims during a public health emergency) and to help rebuild the basic infrastructure necessary to protect the public's health. This article identifies issues in the role of public health nurses in bioterrorism preparedness.

This project was supported under a cooperative agreement from the Centers for Disease Control and Prevention through the Association of Schools of Public Health (ASPH). Grant Number A1023-21/21.

*Corresponding author for proof and reprints. E-mail address: rrowney@umich.edu (R. Rowney).

0029-6465/05/$ – see front matter
doi:10.1016/j.cnur.2005.04.005

ISSUES IN PREPARING FOR BIOTERRORISM
Lack of experience
Bioterrorism threatens national security when large, susceptible populations deliberately are exposed to highly virulent organisms that produce widespread illness. The ability of terrorists to disrupt health care services was seen when unsuspecting victims intentionally were exposed to anthrax in the United States in the fall of 2001. Before that time, anthrax had been considered as the exotic wool-sorters disease [3]. Multiple victims were exposed, and several agencies responded. The agencies were unable to delineate their roles and the responsibilities of each partner. There was not a clear understanding of the chain of command, how to communicate specialized knowledge, or communicate through the media to the general public. Public health officials had difficulty identifying the limits of their own knowledge, authority, and responsibility. In the midst of the chaos, public health nurses were asked to conduct communicable disease investigations, perform clinical tasks, administer mass medication clinics, and communicate with the worried well.

Terminology
The confusion regarding bioterrorism is caused somewhat by terminology. Terms such as disasters, mass casualty incidents, terrorism, and bioterrorism sometimes are used interchangeably. Although there are similarities between the four terms, there are important differences, and Table 1 provides an overview. Veenema describes a disaster as an event that occurs suddenly, causes damage that exceeds the capacity of the responders, and requires outside help. The causes of a disaster are described as nature, equipment malfunction, human error, biological hazards, and disease [4].

The International Nursing Coalition for Mass Casualty Education (INCMCE) was "organized to facilitate the systematic development of sustainable and scalable educational policies related to mass casualty events" [5]. INCMCE emphasizes that a mass casualty event exceeds the day-to-day operational ability of the local responders and compels planners to provide for surge capacity [5].

Terrorism has additional dimensions not specifically seen in the definitions of disaster and mass casualty incidents. Levy and Sidel [1] emphasize that terrorism is politically motivated and intentionally directed toward civilians. Terrorists use the threat or actual act of violence, such as biological, chemical, incendiary, explosive, or nuclear agents as a weapon to instill fear. Bioterrorism frequently is used colloquially to describe all weapons of mass destruction (WMD), which sometimes are referred to as chemical, biological, radiological, nuclear, and explosive (CBRNE) or biological, nuclear, incendiary, chemical, and explosive (BNICE).

Nature of bioterrorism
The nature of a bioterrorist event is like other types of terrorist events in intent but different in terms of agent and timing of events. Bioterrorism creates real or potential victims in a civilian population who fear contracting or dying from

Table 1
Comparison of terms related to bioterrorism

Term	Caused by	Characteristics	Examples
Disaster [4] Sudden event	Nature Equipment failure Human error Biological hazard Disease	Exceeds capacity Causes damage Ecological Loss of life	Earthquake, floods, fire, hurricane Hazardous materials spill Air crash Epidemic Civil strife
Mass Casualty [5] Single event	Natural forces Infrastructure failure Conduct of people	Significant disruption of health and safety Exceeds capability	Hurricane, tornado Plane crash Power outage Terrorist attack Act of war
Terrorism [1] Violence, force	Political motivation	Overwhelms capacity Against civilians Instills fear Crime	May involve weapons of mass destruction (CBRNE) Cyber-terrorism, agro-terrorism and eco terrorism
Bioterrorism [1] Violence, force—may emerge slowly	Political motivation	Against civilians Instill fear Crime	Bioagents

a serious communicable disease [1]. The most effective bioterrorism agent is a biological organism that is highly communicable from person to person and can cause high morbidity and mortality. Infectious diseases caused by a bioterrorist organism are not like a naturally occurring acute event (eg, varicella) that is relatively time-limited. Instead, an intentionally released agent will appear as an index case, then spread to close and secondary contacts over an extended period of time. It is the terrorist's intent is to instill anxiety during large outbreaks of disease and death that evolve slowly over time.

THE ROLE OF PUBLIC HEALTH NURSES IN BIOTERRORISM
Public health nurses who work in a local or state health department are actively involved in all phases of planning, detecting, controlling and responding to an outbreak caused by a bioterrorist agent. Unlike most acute care clinicians who specialize in the care of certain disorders, the scope of the public health nurses' practice can extend from pre-disaster planning, to delivering care during an event, to post-disaster evaluation. Public health nurses are accustomed to handling outbreaks of communicable disease and routinely collaborate with other health care workers in primary care and hospital settings. If an incident is

suspected bioterrorism, the case will involve working with local and federal law enforcement agencies conducting a criminal investigation. Bioterrorism will generate media coverage and a nationwide scare.

Local planning

Local public health departments should have an emergency management coordinator who is responsible for emergency and disaster planning. Local resources are necessary, because a community needs to be able to initiate and sustain its own local response for the first 48 hours following a disaster. It takes time to mobilize distant resources, and how a community responds within those first hours will affect the overall morbidity and mortality associated with the incident [6]. The local coordinator works with law enforcement, emergency management, medical care systems, and public health agencies to ensure a quick and comprehensive response can be provided until state and federal help arrives.

Public health agencies need established relationships with other local agencies to effectively plan and respond to an event. Common wisdom suggests that emergency preparedness partners do not want to meet for the first time while an actual bioterrorism event is unfolding. While working together, the agencies create plans, conduct exercises, and practice drills to build the trust and relationships that will be needed in the first hours and over the long term. Local agencies will need to be able to continue to work together post disaster to provide follow-up and remediation after state and federal agencies retreat from a community.

In order for a public health agency to fulfill its role in a bioterrorism event, whether it is in the lead, collaborative, or secondary/supportive role, all staff must be competent to carry out individual responsibilities [7]. Nurses represent the largest single professional group practicing public health, and they have considerable knowledge of resources in a local community. They are grounded in population-based health practice for individuals, families, groups, and communities. Public health nurses work within three sets of competencies to better prepare for their responsibilities.

Competencies

"A competency is a complex combination of knowledge, skills, and abilities demonstrated by organization members that are critical to the effective and efficient function of the organization" [7]. The three sets of competencies relevant to the public health nurse to prepare for bioterrorism and emergency preparedness are core competencies, public health nursing competencies, and specific bioterrorism and emergency preparedness competencies [7–9]. The bioterrorism competencies include specialty knowledge, skills, and attitudes that flow from the public health nursing competencies that flow from the original core competencies identified for all public health workers (Fig. 1).

The Council on Linkages between Academia and Public Health Practice identified core competencies that encompass eight domains for all public health

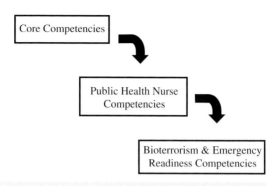

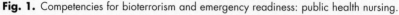

Fig. 1. Competencies for bioterrorism and emergency readiness: public health nursing.

professionals, not just public health nurses. These domains of core competencies are:

- Analytic assessment skills
- Basic public health sciences
- Cultural competency
- Communications
- Community dimensions of practice
- Financial management
- Leadership and systems thinking
- Policy development/program planning

The Quad Council of Public Health Nursing Organizations is an alliance of four national nursing organizations that address public health nursing issues. The members include the Association of Community Health Nurse Educators, American Nurses Association, American Public Health Association Public Health Nursing Section, and the Association of State and Territorial Directors of Nursing. The council developed a list of public health nursing competencies that flowed from most of the domains identified within the original core competencies. Although most of the public health nurse competencies relate tangentially to bioterrorism and emergency preparedness, the most specific for public health nurses reads, "prepares and implements emergency response plan" [9].

The Centers for Disease Control and Prevention (CDC) have endorsed competencies for public health clinical staff and defined the roles for public health nurses [7]. The purpose of the competencies is to assure workforce readiness for bioterrorism and emergency preparedness. The CDC also have established competency-based training in schools of public health through a network of centers for public health preparedness. The mission of the network, in partnership with state and local public health departments, is to provide training for the public health workforce. Competency-based training promotes the public health nurse's ability to master the behaviors necessary to execute the role in the event of an incident.

Roles for public health nursing

The specific role for public health nurses is defined by the bioterrorism and emergency competencies and by the agency preparedness plan where they are employed. Levy and Sidel [1] identified four overall roles for all health professionals in terrorism and public health. These are: (1) develop improved preparedness, (2) respond to the health consequences of terrorist acts and threats, (3) take action to prevent terrorism, and (4) promote a balance between response to terrorism and other public health concerns. These roles can be adapted to nurses working in state and local governmental public health settings by cross-walking with the competency sets.

Develop improved preparedness

Public health departments across the nation are organized around similar missions but have strategically different ways of functioning. These differences are based on structure, funding sources, and the leadership of the organization. Public health leaders set policy and direction and assume overall responsibility for assuring that their agency is prepared for bioterrorism. Public health nurses are active participants in writing, updating, reviewing, and exercising emergency response plans for their agencies. The plan establishes relationships with other partners involved in emergency response and addresses clinical protocols, surge capacity, and safety measures needed in the event of an actual occurrence [7].

A critical competency for all is knowledge of the chain of command. Public health professionals have adopted the incident command system used by the military, law enforcement, and fire fighters for use in bioterrorism and emergency preparedness. Also known as the incident management system, this system provides a common organizational structure and terminology, integrated communications, and consolidated action plans to protect life, property, and the environment [10].

The public health nurses' functional role is outlined in their agency's plan. Nurses are expected to seek out training and identify key system resources to assure effective preparedness to meet the responsibilities identified in the plan. Staff nurses, supervisors, and nurse administrators are educated before an event to be better able to communicate accurate information to clients, media, the general public, and other health professionals. Continuing education about the clinical manifestations of biological agents can be obtained readily through print and online sources [11–13]. For example, the CDC has categorized biological agents according to accessibility, ease of use, potential for social disruption, morbidity, and mortality [11]. Category A, B. and C agents result in diseases not normally seen in everyday public health practice, and the very mention of names such as smallpox, anthrax, and plague raises grave concerns among the public. Nurses are among the most trusted and accessible of all health professionals. Therefore, family, friends, neighbors, patients, and clients frequently ask a nurse for health information about emerging infectious diseases and bioterrorism. The nurse can use or refer the lay public to fact sheets on biological agents that are available through the CDC [13]. The goal is to help the public to become educated, follow a rational response, and avoid false information that could cause panic.

Public health nurses are responsible for obtaining and sending biological and chemical specimens for laboratory analysis, and nurses need access to updated information. Biological analysis is coordinated through the national public health laboratory system, which was developed to promote effective working relationships between clinical and public health laboratories and to strengthen the country's ability to test for all types of biological agents. Each biosafety-level laboratory performs a different function [14], and clinicians must be aware of the different requirements for each type of agent and specimen.

In contrast, the chemical laboratory program is being developed across the nation, and testing for chemical metabolites associated with chemical terrorism is not as advanced as for biological agents. The chemical laboratory network consists of different levels of laboratories with roles similar to those for biological testing. In the case of a suspected terrorist event, chemical specimens would be considered as criminal and forensic evidence and would need to have a documented chain of custody. Public health agencies need education regarding creating a chain of custody, the forms to use, and how each agency retains its own written document to assure continuous accountability.

Respond to health consequences

The public health nurse's functional role in bioterrorism is outlined by each agency; however, a need remains to allow for creative problem solving and flexible thinking [5]. An act of bioterrorism is difficult to identify early, because biological agents cause diseases that present with symptoms similar to common illnesses such as influenza [11]. An astute physician or nurse will likely be the first to recognize an unusual illness. He or she will need to diagnose and quickly report suspected cases immediately to public health and law enforcement authorities.

Public health nurses are active in the epidemiology and surveillance functions of public health agencies and participate in disease outbreak investigations. Because nurses identify and interview persons potentially exposed to bioterrorism agents, they need to know the signs and symptoms of all suspected diseases. They will assess, triage, isolate, treat, and provide public health support for victims and responders [5]. Many plans call for public health nurses to staff mass clinics to dispense vaccines, antimicrobials, and antitoxins made available through local sources or the CDC's Strategic National Stockpile. Other plans deploy public health nurses to assist with shelters, schools, or places with other vulnerable populations.

In the event of a suspected bioterrorist event, a community can provide medical resources through the Modular Emergency Medical System (MEMS). The MEMS model directs people away from overcrowded emergency departments to satellite community-based centers that triage, treat, and give supportive care. The centers are called acute care centers and are designed to relieve the overcrowding of hospitals and other acute care clinics. The MEMS model includes neighborhood emergency help centers and a community outreach component. Public health nurses may be asked to staff the neighborhood emergency help centers and community outreach centers to triage, give prophylaxis, refer to resources, and give self-help information [15].

Regardless of the setting, the public health nurse must be competent to respond to the psychological impact of a bioterrorism event for the victims, the public, and the workers responding to the event [5]. The psychosocial impact was documented for the Sept. 11, 2001, attacks and the anthrax incidents that occurred later that same year [16]. Taintor states, "the mental health of the population is a prime target of terrorists" [17].

Bioterrorism response plans should include reviewing practitioners' teaching and counseling skills and how to help victims who need emotional support. Public health nurses work with vulnerable populations and are acquainted with children, families, and communities at high risk for psychosocial difficulties. In a disaster, even normal-functioning individuals may experience problems directly related to the disaster [18]. Nurses need to be able to recognize the signs and symptoms of human stress responses (ie, acute stress reactions or post-traumatic stress disorder), anxiety, depression, fear, and grief and be able to make referrals to the appropriate resources for care [19]. Nurses may be involved in more structured programs, such as critical incident stress management teams or become specifically trained in peer-to-peer counseling [20]. Nurses must be cautious not to overextend themselves and ignore their own physical and mental health needs. The excitement and adrenalin involved in the initial quick response is replaced by exhaustion over the long term. An incident of biological terrorism will require a sustained effort on the part of the public health workforce.

Take action to prevent terrorism

Public health agencies are responsible for ensuring the safety of the general public by preventing communicable diseases. Nurses routinely conduct screening activities and provide anti-infective medications and immunizations to susceptible populations. Although the ideal biological weapon is an organism that does not have a means of preventing or effective treatment, there are highly virulent agents that have been used, despite a vaccine being available. Smallpox would pose a significant threat to public health in the United States, because the general population is virtually unvaccinated and thus unprotected. The smallpox threat has received considerable national attention [21], and a major health care initiative was launched in late 2002 to vaccinate a core group of health care workers and emergency response personnel. The intent of vaccinating this group is to develop a work force that could respond to suspected cases.

Most nurses have limited or no clinical experience with the smallpox vaccine, its administration, and adverse reactions. As public health agencies develop smallpox preparedness plans, additional nurses will need to be vaccinated so they can administer the vaccine in massive vaccination clinics. All nurses are challenged to become familiar with the disease, the vaccine, and the method of administration as part of a nationwide smallpox preparation initiative.

Other potentially lethal diseases also have vaccines available. Anthrax can be prevented if vaccine is given pre-exposure. Unfortunately, the safety of the vaccine came into question after it was mandated for members of the US military, and there is ongoing research on the product [12].

Influenza vaccine seldom is considered as part of the bioterrorism and emergency preparedness prevention efforts; however, preventing the disease has added benefits. Illnesses caused by bioterrorism agents can present with signs and symptoms similar to influenza. Immunizations should be encouraged to reduce the background incidence of influenza that could mask the diagnosis and early identification of a more serious bioterrorist attack. Public health nurses currently conduct massive community influenza immunization clinics that contribute to developing the herd immunity of a population at risk.

A long-term goal for all health care clinicians to prevent bioterrorism is to reduce access to potential bioterrorist agents [1]. The security of public health and research laboratories has been strengthened since the anthrax events, and all health care providers should be aware of and follow the stringent federal guidelines and regulations for laboratory security [14]. Another long-term effort is to advocate for the control, reduction, and elimination of WMDs. Several countries, including the United States, have developed, produced, and tested biological weapons. The history of their use is a sobering chronicle of how science and technology can be counterproductive to the ideals of nursing and public health [1,22].

Promote a balance

Public health nurses are on the front lines of delivering community-focused, population-based services. Daily, nurses find that they must balance several priorities and competing demands, such as undoing health disparities; providing care for the uninsured; and treating the chronic effects of obesity, tobacco, drugs, infectious diseases, violence, and injury control [22]. Now the new efforts to combat bioterrorism have presented a paradox for many clinicians.

The CDC, under the direction of national and state public health policy makers, has invested considerable resources into state and local health departments to improve bioterrorism preparedness. Money has been allocated to bolster the capacity for epidemiology, laboratory services, training, communications, and planning functions. The efforts to improve the infrastructure created for bioterrorism and emergency readiness already have shown their usefulness for response to other public health problems, such as West Nile virus, SARS, and other infectious disease outbreaks. Unfortunately, the new resources also have been viewed as a distraction from addressing other urgent problems that require the attention of public health. State and local health departments are subject to increased scrutiny by policy makers to use the money wisely to address bioterrorism and emergency preparedness [23] and must not risk using the new money to supplant funding in areas where support has been decreased. Public health providers will struggle with how to use the resulting products to support other aspects of population-based interventions without violating the original intent of the investment.

Public health nurses provide further balance to bioterrorism preparedness programs by evaluating the effectiveness, accessibility, and quality of public health services [24]. Well-designed studies are needed to test a plan, clarify the nurse's role, improve coordination and communication, identify gaps in resources, and provide an opportunity for improvement. One study [25] evaluated emergency preparedness training and perceived barriers for public health nurses to work during a public health emergency. The study concluded that the training was useful; however, nurses needed to better balance their personal and professional lives and to develop disaster plans for their home, family, workplace and community. Anyone can become a disaster victim and will have to face competing personal and professional responsibilities [25,26]. Resources, such as the American Red Cross and the Federal Emergency Management Agency (FEMA), have made information easily available for individuals to access and tailor for their own personal preparation for any kind of disaster.

SUMMARY

Recent terrorist events in the United States have accentuated the role of public health nurses as first responders in bioterrorism incidents. Diseases caused by a bioterrorist agent are not likely to be detected and will evolve slowly over time, taxing the resources of local public health agencies. Because their role is competency-based, public health nurses participate in disease prevention efforts, such as providing immunizations, identifying new cases by signs and symptoms, and participating in disease investigations. If a bioterrorism event is suspected, nurses work within agency plans and established chains of command to staff outreach sites, conduct mass clinics, promote responsible communications, and provide teaching and psychosocial support. Nurses also continually re-evaluate their role and performance by participating in exercises and drills, and they extend the planning to their personal lives also.

References

[1] Levy BS, Sidel VW. Challenges that terrorism poses to public health. In: Levy BS, Sidel VW, editors. Terrorism and public health, a balanced approach to strengthening systems and protecting people. New York: Oxford University Press; 2003.

[2] Gebbie KM. Holding society, and nursing, together. Am J Nurs 2002;102:73.

[3] Benenson A. Control of communicable diseases manual. 16th edition. Washington (DC): American Public Health Association; 1995.

[4] Veenema TG. Disaster nursing and emergency preparedness for chemical biological and radiological terrorism and other hazards. New York: Springer Publishing Company; 2003.

[5] International Nursing Coalition for Mass Casualty Education. International nursing coalition for mass casualty education mission statement. Available from: http://www.mc.vanderbilt.edu/nursing/coalitions/INCMCE/missnstmnt.pdf-7.5KB. Accessed March 19, 2004.

[6] Geberding JL, Hughes JM, Kooplan JP. Bioterrorism preparedness and response: clinicians and public health agencies as essential partners. In: Henderson D, Inglesby TV, O'Toole T, editors. Bioterrorism: guidelines for medical and public health management. Chicago: AMA; 2002.

[7] Columbia University School of Nursing Center for Health Policy. Bioterrorism and emergency readiness competencies for all public health workers. Atlanta (GA): Centers for Disease Control and Prevention; 2002.

[8] Council on Linkages Between Academia and Public Health Practice. Core competencies for public health professionals. Washington (DC): Public Health Foundation; 2001.

[9] Quad Council of Public Health Nursing Organizations. Core competencies for public health nurses, a project of the council on linkages between academia and public health practice funded by the Health Resources and Services Administration, 2003.

[10] Johnson M. Incident management system local and state public health agencies. Proceedings of Michigan Department of Community Health training on incident management. Lansing (MI): Michigan Department of Community Health; 2002.

[11] Weinstein RS, Alibek K. Biological and chemical terrorism, a guide for healthcare providers and first responders. New York: Thieme Medical; 2003.

[12] Henderson D, Inglesby T, O'Toole T. Bioterrorism guidelines for medical and public health management. Chicago: American Medical Association; 2002.

[13] Centers for Disease Control and Prevention. Bioterrorism agents/diseases. Available from: http://www.bt.cdc.gov/agent/agentlist.asp. Accessed March 20, 2004.

[14] Centers for Disease Control and Prevention. Laboratory security and emergency response guidance for laboratories working with select agents. MMWR 2002;51(No. RR-19).

[15] Church J, Skidmore S. Modular emergency medical system (MEMS): how's it going? Proceedings of Michigan Department of Community Health, Office of Public Health Preparedness on Challenging our Assumptions. Lansing (MI): Michigan Department of Community Health; 2003.

[16] Allds M, Ludwick R. One year later: the impact and aftermath of September 11. Available at: http://www.nursingworld.org/ojin/topic19/tpc19lnx.htm. Accessed September 18, 2003.

[17] Taintor Z. Addressing mental health needs. In: Levy BS, Sidel VW, editors. Terrorism and public health: a balanced approach to strengthening systems and protecting people. New York: Oxford University Press, Incorporated; 2003.

[18] Gordon NS, Farberow NL, Maida CA. Children and disasters. Philadelphia: Taylor & Francis; 1999.

[19] Haggerty B, Williams RA. Psychosocial issues related to bioterrorism for nurses subcompetencies. Presented at the University of Michigan Academic Center for Public Health Preparedness. Ann Arbor (MI), September 15, 2003.

[20] Antai-Otong D. Critical incident stress debriefing: a health promotion model for workplace violence. Perspect Psychiatr Care 2001;37:125.

[21] Agency for Healthcare Research and Quality. Addressing the smallpox threat: issues, strategies and tools. Available at: http://www.ahrq.gov/news/ulp/btbriefs/btbrief1.htm. Accessed March 16, 2004.

[22] Berkowitz B. Public health nursing practice: aftermath of September 11, 2001. Online Journal of Issues in Nursing 2002;7:11.

[23] Frist B. Public health and national security: the critical role of increased federal support. Health Aff 2002;21:117.

[24] Gebbie KM. Emergency and disaster preparedness: core competencies for nurses: what every nurse should but may not know. Am J Nurs 2002;102:46.

[25] Qureshi K, Merrill J, Gershon R, et al. Emergency preparedness training for public health nurses: a pilot study. J Urban Health 2002;79:413.

[26] Silva MC, Ludwick R. Ethics and terrorism: September 11, 2001, and its aftermath. Online Journal of Issues in Nursing 2003;8:5.

Nurs Clin N Am 40 (2005) 511–521

NURSING CLINICS
OF NORTH AMERICA

LSEVIER
AUNDERS

The Role of the Nurse Practitioner in Disaster Planning and Response

Frank L. Cole, PhD, RN, CEN, CS, FNP, FAAN

Department of Acute and Continuing Care; Emergency Nurse Practitioner Education;
The University of Texas Health Science Center at Houston, 6901 Bertner Avenue,
Room 697, Houston, TX 77030, USA

Tropical storm Allison ravaged Houston and surrounding areas from June 5 through 9, 2001. The storm produced record levels of rainfall, with nearly 37 inches of rain in one area of the city [1]. The rain and flooding affected the Texas Medical Center, causing power outages and disruption of normal functioning. There was no access into or out of the medical center area; communications were lost with outside agencies, and there was a need to evacuate patients who were on life support equipment. The entire nursing staff of the Texas Medical Center found themselves as disaster care providers [2].

All disasters are unique, but the tropical storm demonstrated that all nurses can have key roles in disaster response. In the past, "disaster management was seen as specialty training for nurses in emergency rooms, pubic health, and the military" [3]. This has changed since the Joint Commission on Accreditation of Hospital Organizations (JCAHO) began to mandate that hospital-based nurses participate in biannual disaster drills.

The role of advanced practice nurses (APNs), including nurse practitioners (NPs), in disaster planning and response is not defined well. Although APNs and NPs have provided health care services during disasters, little appears in the literature about their role. This oversight becomes more important in a national disaster, as APNs and NPs represent a significant portion of the nursing workforce. According to the American Academy of Nurse Practitioners (AAPN), in 2004 there were over 106,000 NPs in the United States [4]. This article focuses on critical factors to consider when preparing and planning NPs within a community's disaster response.

PREPARING NURSE PRACTITIONERS FOR DISASTER RESPONSE
Nurse practitioners are prepared in several different graduate-level educational settings. Of the NPs listed in the AAPN 2004 database, 88% held a graduate degree, and 92% had a national certification [4]. The NP role was developed

E-mail address: frank.l.cole@uth.tmc.edu

0029-6465/05/$ – see front matter
doi:10.1016/j.cnur.2005.04.007

in 1965 by Loretta Ford at the University of Colorado. The first NPs focused on improving health care for children, and graduates of this program were considered as pediatric NPs [5]. Over time, the role of NPs has expanded to family nurse practitioner (FNP), adult nurse practitioner (ANP), and gerontological nurse practitioner (GNP). These programs focused on primary care [6].

The scope of NP practice has been extended to acute and critical care settings [7–8], including emergency care [9]. Graduates of acute and emergency care NP programs provide: care to more acutely ill individuals, including those with life-threatening conditions; life-saving treatments; and invasive diagnostic and therapeutic interventions. Additionally, NPs who provide care in emergency settings often have procedural skills that their counterparts may not possess [10] (Box 1).

Educational prerequisites

Applicants to graduate NP programs are required to have a Bachelor of Science degree in nursing and 1 or more years of nursing experience related to their specialty area. Most NPs have substantially more than 1 year of nursing experience before enrolling. A study of NPs found that those who practice in emergency care settings had an average of 13.77 years (SD = 7.55) of experience before becoming an NP [11]. In a similar study, NPs in emergency care had worked as registered nurses (RNs) for an average of 17.9 years (SD = 6.7) but had worked as NPs only an average of 5.2 years (SD = 5.0) [10].

The many years of nursing experience that students bring to the NP educational program helps to shape their practice after graduation. Because of a low number of emergency NP programs in the United States, many emergency nurses opt to attend a primary care program where they learn primary care management. In practice, this knowledge is tempered by their years of practical emergency care experience. For example, a patient with a group A beta hemolytic streptococci throat infection would be prescribed an oral antibiotic in a primary care setting. In the emergency department, the patient would most likely be given an intramuscular injection of an appropriate antibiotic because for financial or personal issues, many patients who seek care in an emergency department do not follow-up with filling prescriptions or seeing primary care practitioners. This example demonstrates how NPs from different educational and clinical backgrounds may bring unique knowledge and skills to a disaster situation.

Educational standards for disaster care
Core competencies

Core competencies have been identified for registered nurses in disasters [12] (Box 2); however, no such competencies exist for APNs or NPs. It is possible that because the NP is also an RN, that the basic RN competencies will serve as a minimum for the NP. This issue still needs to be defined. Since the original competencies were developed, the American Medical Association has

Box 1: Procedures performed by 50% or more of the nurse practitioners in emergency care

Use fluorescein staining

Remove a foreign body of the eye

Interpret 12 lead electrocardiogram

Perform a single-layer closure of an extremity or trunk wound

Remove a foreign body from soft tissues

Perform digital nerve blocks

Splint extremities

Pack wounds

Inject local anesthetics

Incise and drain an abscess

Close lacerations on the face

Perform staple closure of wound

Debride burns

Interpret arterial blood gases

Perform nail trephination

Remove finger or toe nail(s)

Reduce dislocations

Revise a wound for closure

Clinically clear cervical spine

Perform a multiple-layer wound closure

Perform a slit lamp examination

Reduce fractures of small bones (eg, finger)

Perform a nail bed closure

Insert a drain into a wound

Remove fecal impactions

Insert nasal packing

Radiographically clear cervical spine

Order/administer conscious sedation

Perform an arthrocentesis

Dilate eye(s)

Perform tonometry

Insert a drain into a Bartholin's cyst

Insert an anoscope

Perform a sexual assault exam

Incise thrombosed hemorrhoids

Box 2: Core disaster competencies for nurses as identified by Gebbie and Qureshi

Describe the agency's role in responding to a range of emergencies that might arise.

Describe the chain of command in emergency response.

Identify and locate the agency's emergency response plan (or the pertinent portion of it).

Describe emergency response functions or roles and demonstrate them in regularly performed drills.

Demonstrate the use of equipment (including personal protective equipment) and the skills required in emergency response during regular drills.

Demonstrate the correct operation of all equipment used for emergency communication.

Describe communication roles in emergency response (1) within your agency, (2) with news media, (3) with the general public (including patients and families), and (4) with personal contacts (one's own family, friends, and neighbors).

Identify the limits of your own knowledge, skills, and authority, and identify key system resources for referring matters that exceed these limits.

Apply creative problem-solving skills and flexible thinking to the situation, within the confines of your role, and evaluate the effectiveness of all actions taken.

Recognize deviations from the norm that might indicate an emergency and describe appropriate action.

Participate in continuing education to maintain up-to-date knowledge in relevant areas.

Participate in evaluating every drill or response and identify necessary changes to the plan.

From Gebbie KM, Qureshi K. Emergency and disaster preparedness: core competencies for nurses. Am J Nursing 2002;102:46–51; with permission.

partnered with others to develop the National Disaster Life Support (NDLS) program, with the goal of standardizing and strengthening emergency response training in the area of disasters [13]. The NDLS consists of three courses: core disaster life support, basic disaster life support, and advanced disaster life support; these courses are open to nurses [13].

Disaster educational content

Some NP educational programs may have information about disaster care or the ability of the NP to provide health care services during a disaster. At the time of this publication, there is no published educational standard regarding core knowledge of disasters and management of mass casualty patients for NP students. Until more structured courses are made available during initial training, NPs can enroll in NDLS courses and use continuing education resources, such as The Virtual Naval Hospital (http://www.vnh.org/), which contains links to other sources, such as First Aid for Soldiers, GMO Manual, Standard First Aid Course, and the Iowa Family Practice Handbook. Another source is the Textbook of Military Medicine: Medical Aspects of Chemical and Biological Warfare (http://www.vnh.org/MedAspChemBioWar/index.html), which provides clinical information about toxic agents and decontamination. Information about decontamination can also be found in the Textbook of Military Medicine: Medical Aspects of Chemical and Biological Warfare (http://www.vnh.org/MedAsp-ChemBioWar/index.html). Alternately, information on decontamination of ambulatory and nonambulatory patients can be found at the Hazmat for Health care Web site (http://www.hazmatforhealthcare.org/download/doc/misc/Patient_Decontamination_Procedure-complete.doc).

PLANNING FOR NURSE PRACTITIONERS' RESPONSE IN DISASTERS

Practice acts

Registered nurses

Registered nurses frequently want to answer a call for help during a disaster but run into problems with licensure in other states. This issue has been addressed partially by cooperative legislation between states that belong to the Nurse Licensure Compact (Box 3) [14]. RNs with licensure in any compact state are allowed to practice in other compact states without first obtaining licensure in those other states [15]. During nondisaster situations, RNs who are licensed in a noncompact state will not be allowed to practice in another state without first gaining permission from the new state's nursing board. RNs who wish to volunteer in another state during a disaster should determine if their state is a member in the nursing licensure compact and bring their nursing license as proof.

Certain states have adapted legislation that addresses licensure limitations during disasters. "The New York State Nurse Practice Act contains an exemption for federal, state, and civil emergencies. During such emergencies, RNs need not be licensed in New York State, but must bring with them evidence of current licensure in another state" [16]. During the 2001 World Trade Center disaster, the National Guard precluded nurses from entering the disaster area if they did not have a valid nursing license [16].

Nurse practitioners

Nurse practitioners receive their license to function as APNs by applying and being approved by their home state board of nursing. The board of nursing delineates the scope of practice of the NP according to the state's nurse practice act and specifies the legal authority for what a nurse may do in that state [17]. All but a few states require that the NP practice in a collaborative or supervising relationship with a physician who must be available for consultation. Because there is no distinction made regarding how the NP would function during a disaster, the NP needs to negotiate specific operating procedures if the physician collaborator is not immediately available. NPs who practice at

Box 3: States that have implemented the registered nurse licensure compact as of March 2005

Arizona
Arkansas
Delaware
Idaho
Iowa
Maine
Maryland
Mississippi
Nebraska
New Mexico
North Carolina
North Dakota
South Dakota
Tennessee
Texas
Utah
Virginia
Wisconsin

a distance from the physician or who want to work within another state likely will encounter licensing restrictions.

Currently, a NP can practice only in a state in which he or she has prior approval. The nurse licensure compact only has recently addressed NPs [18] but the only state to pass this compact as of March 7, 2005, was Utah [15].

In a disaster, North Carolina's Board of Nursing rules for NPs states "a nurse practitioner approved to practice in this state or another state may perform medical acts, as a nurse practitioner under the supervision of a physician licensed to practice medicine in North Carolina during a disaster in a county in which a state of disaster has been declared or counties contiguous to a county in which a state of disaster has been declared" [19]. The NP is required to notify the Medical and Nursing Boards within 15 days of first performing medical acts. Additionally the document states that "teams of physician(s) and nurse practitioner(s) practicing pursuant to this rule shall not be required to maintain on-site documentation describing supervisory arrangements and instructions for prescriptive authority as otherwise required" [19].

Medical liability and malpractice

Nurse practitioners need to assess their risk for medical liability and determine if they have malpractice insurance coverage if they practice in a disaster away from their usual place of employment. Connecticut has enacted a statue that declares NPs, physician assistants, and physician civil defense employees when the governor declares a state of emergency, and this removes the concern about insurance coverage [20].

Because all NPs are RNs, there is a question if the NP could choose to function only as a RN during a disaster. Herrick provides a thorough discussion of NPs who function in the RN versus NP role, and unfortunately, there is no clear-cut answer as to which role to assume in a disaster situation [21].

Phases of a disaster

Disaster researchers and managers have attempted to define disasters in terms of phases. This process allows a systematic way to plan and evaluate responses. For the purpose of this discussion, the NP's role during a disaster can include:

- Preparation phase: assessment of personal and community risk and abilities to respond
- Mitigation phase: use of warning systems to alert endangered people to take appropriate action
- Response phase: initiating life-saving and illness/injury prevention interventions
- Recover phase: mobilizing community to rebuild short- and long-term projects

Preparation

Education

Nurse practitioners should help develop disaster plans in their family, work setting and community. NPs are a valuable source of information regarding nursing and medical care; needs of ill or injured individuals; and types of medical equipment, medications, and other supplies that will be needed during a disaster. The NP can help teach emergency responders assessment skills, extremity splinting, wound care, application of dressings, and other first aid skills. NPs should ensure that plans include meeting the psychological needs of victims and rescue personnel.

Nurse practitioners may work with individuals who are new to an area and do not have prior knowledge of local risks. In their day-to-day practice, or as a community outreach effort, NPs can review the importance of personal disaster preparedness, significance of community safety programs, how to interpret warning systems, and how individuals should respond if warnings are issued. They can discuss emergency supplies (eg, drinking water, flashlights, batteries, and a portable radio), how to stock and use first aid, and the location of community resources such as hurricane shelters.

Modeling preparedness

Nurse practitioners should assemble emergency supplies, study evacuation or shelter options, and create a plan with their own family members. The plan should cover specific issues, such as how to communicate with each other if they are separated during a disaster, where to meet, or the telephone number of a family member or friend in another geographical area that everyone can call to report his or her whereabouts. Family members should be encouraged to practice the plan.

Mitigation phase

When there is warning of an impending disaster, NPs need to follow the disaster plan at their place of employment and implement their family plan. NPs may be given any type of role, depending on the facility and the other health care providers available. The roles can range from triage to assessing patients for discharge or transfer.

Response phase

Changes in standard operations

Nurse practitioners can use the experience of others to implement changes in operation during a disaster. Newberry recommends the use of a tracking system and protocols for handling telephone calls and off-duty employees [22].

A chain-of-evidence document can be used to track patient movement through an agency or institution. The document records the patient's location each time he or she is moved and provides a means of identifying where any patient is at any time. This same method can be used to identify which patients need decontamination [22].

Telephone calls add to the chaos and can be disruptive to any system during a crisis. Newberry [22] recommends a policy and procedure that limits staff time with calls. Once a disaster occurs, staff members are encouraged to make one essential telephone call to contact family and remind family members of the importance of refraining from calling. One staff person then is assigned to answer all incoming telephone calls, logging the call, and telling the caller that someone will return the call when possible. Only critical calls are transferred [22].

During a disaster, many off-duty personnel respond to the agency to offer assistance. This practice can result in a large number of staff available initially but not long-term. Newberry suggests that management assess the ongoing need for staff and call in individuals when needed [22].

Temporary clinics

Nurse practitioners may be involved in establishing temporary clinics or other settings in which health care can be delivered. During the 2002 Hayman fire in Castle Rock, Colo., an NP provided medical assistance out of a trailer while the fire was still being fought. (Barbara Kurlan, MSN, RN, FNP, personnel communication, March 5, 2004). She indicated that the complexity of problems ranged from prevention to a grand mal seizure, and her role involved dispensing over-the-counter medications; providing health care education; addressing issues concerning foot care; and managing lacerations, orthopedic injuries, dehydration, respiratory ailments, and eye injuries. Her role involved triage and evacuation of critically injured personnel.

During a disaster, power outages and communication disruptions are common; therefore NPs need to have resources on hand and to be able to function with previously established medical directives. NPs may be asked to care for victims, rescue and reconstruction workers. At the same time, all health care providers should be aware of potential toxic agents that may not produce illness for several days [23]. NPs need to maintain a high risk of suspicion after a disaster and participate in identifying and reporting symptoms to public health officials who are conducting syndromic surveillance (ie, process that collects widespread data in an attempt to identify early signs of a major outbreak).

Psychiatric NPs can help victims and rescue workers cope with the psychological consequences of the disaster. After the 2001 World Trade Center disaster, one NP helped set up a treatment center that managed patients with hyperventilation, anxiety attacks, fractures, hyper-reactive airways, and minor injuries [24]. At the same time, psychiatric NPs counseled survivors of the attack and relatives of the victims [24].

Recovery
Working with the effects of stress
Nurse practitioners need to be alert to the consequences of stress following a disaster and refer survivors and workers who may experience stress disorders. Potential long-term stress disorders are characterized by symptom clusters that include re-experiencing the event, avoidance or numbing behaviors, and increased physiologic arousal [25]. NPs followed high school adolescents after Hurricane Hugo (occurred in 1989). Out of 507 students, 63 were found to exhibit symptoms of psychological distress, and 27 required evaluation by a nurse psychotherapist [26]. Students were found to have adjustment reaction, depression, post-traumatic stress disorder, or serious family problems [26].

Stress following a disaster may manifest itself in other ways. Curtis and colleagues investigated changes in reports and incidence of child abuse following natural disasters [27]. They found that child abuse increased after Hurricane Hugo in South Carolina and the Loma Prieta earthquake in California. Gay noted significant increases in violence (eg, gunshot wounds, assault, and rape) after Hurricane Floyd [28]. Marriage, births, and divorce rates increased in counties declared as disaster areas after Hurricane Hugo [29]. Adults were noted to have increased blood pressure after Mt. St. Helen erupted [30], and adolescents who experienced Hurricane Hugo also were found to have higher blood pressures readings [31].

SUMMARY
Registered nurses have a long history of being involved in disaster planning and response; however, the role of the NP is defined less well. As the number of NPs grows, their role in disaster care will continue to evolve. The major impediments to an expanded role include inconsistent educational preparation, licensure restrictions, pre-established collaboration agreements with physicians, and medical liability. Utah, North Carolina, and Connecticut have provided a model for other states to consider. NPs can contribute to disaster preparedness in all phases of planning and response.

References

[1] National Weather Service Forecast Office. Tropical storm Allison floods, June 5–9, 2001. Available at: http://www.srh.noaa.gov/hgx/projects/allison01.htm. Accessed February 24, 2005.

[2] Sebastian SV, Styron SL, Reize SN, et al. Resiliency of accomplished critical care nurses in a natural disaster. Crit Care Nurse 2003;23:24–36.

[3] Pattillo MM. Mass casualty disaster nursing course. Nurse Educ 2003;28:271–5.

[4] American Academy of Nurse Practitioners. Academy update, December 2004. Available at: http://www.aanp.org/NR/rdonlyres/ehnzpu3qjhas7ttt5alhk3fgit3cb5iepuhu7ogvl jykvs2ntdy5jf6ipbo5amegt3yb53j7fundfj/December20042.pdf. Accessed February 24, 2005.

[5] Ford LC, Silver HK. Expanded role of the nurse in child care. Nurs Outlook 1967;15:43–5.

[6] Hanna DL. The primary care nurse practitioner. In: Hamric AB, Spross JA, Hanson CM, editors. Advanced nursing practice: an integrative approach. 2nd edition. Philadelphia: WB Saunders; 2000. p. 407–24.

[7] Keane A, Richmond T. Tertiary NPs. Image J Nurs Sch 1993;25:281–4.

[8] Keane A, Richmond T, Kaiser L. Critical care nurse practitioners: evolution of the advanced practice nursing role. Am J Crit Care 1994;3:232–7.

[9] Cole FL, Ramirez E. The emergency nurse practitioner: An educational model. J Emerg Nurs 1997;23:112–5.

[10] Cole FL, Ramirez E. Activities and procedures performed by nurse practitioners in emergency care settings. J Emerg Nurs 2000;26:455–63.

[11] Cole FL, Ramirez E. A profile of nurse practitioners in emergency care settings. J Am Acad Nurse Pract 2002;14:183–7.

[12] Gebbie KM, Qureshi K. Emergency and disaster preparedness: Core competencies for nurses. Am J Nurs 2002;102:46–51.

[13] American Medical Association. National disaster life support. Available at: http://www.ama-assn.org/ama/pub/category/12606.html. Accessed March 7, 2005.

[14] National Council of State Boards of Nursing. Nurse licensure compact implementation. Available at: http://www.ncsbn.org/nlc/rnlpvncompact_mutual_recognition_state.asp. Accessed March 7, 2005.

[15] National Council of State Boards of Nursing. Nurse licensure compact. Available at: http://www.ncsbn.org/nlc/index.asp. Accessed March 7, 2005.

[16] Orr ML. Ready or not, disasters happen. Available at: http://www.nursingworld.org/ojin/topic19/tpc19_2.htm. Accessed March 7, 2005.

[17] Rust DH, Magdic KS. The acute care nurse practitioner. In: Hamric AB, Spross JA, Hanson CM, editors. Advanced nursing practice: an integrative approach. 2nd edition. Philadelphia: WB Saunders; 2000. p. 427–35.

[18] National Council of State Boards of Nursing. Advanced practice registered nurse compact. Available at: http://www.ncsbn.org/pdfs/aprncompact.asp. Accessed March 7, 2005.

[19] North Carolina Board of Nursing. 21 NCAC.0814 practicing during a disaster. Available at: http://www.ncbon.com/prac-nprules.asp. Accessed March 7, 2005.

[20] Herrick T. National emergency preparedness: how much progress have we made? Clinical News 2004;8(4):1. 16–8.

[21] Herrick T. What are you liable for? Scope of practice concerns when clinicians filler lesser positions. Clinician News 2002;6(10):17–9.

[22] Newberry L. Practical suggestions for helping emergency nurses handle mass casualties. Disaster Manag Response 2002;1:15–7.

[23] Barajas K, Stewart WA, Combs EW. The Army chemical/biological SMART (Smart-CB) team: The nurse's role. Critical Care Clinics of North America 2003;15:257–64.

[24] Wasserman N. Helpless in tragedy: thousands mobilize to aid wounded, but few survivors emerge. Clinician News 2001;5(9):1. 4–5.

[25] Mitchell AM, Sakraida TJ, Kameg K. Overview of post-traumatic stress. Disaster Manag Response 2002;1:10–4.
[26] Hardin SB, Weinrich S, Weinrich M, et al. Effects of a long-term psychosocial nursing intervention on adolescents exposed to catastrophic stress. Issues Ment Health Nurs 2002; 23:537–51.
[27] Curtis T, Miller BC, Berry EH. Changes in reports and incidence of child abuse following natural disasters. Child Abuse Negl 2000;24:1151–62.
[28] Gay EV. Hurricane Floyd and the ensuing flood in North Carolina: a personal journal. J Emerg Nurs 2002;28:216–22.
[29] Cohan CL, Cole SW. Life course transitions and natural disaster: marriage, birth, and divorce following Hurricane Hugo. J Fam Psychol 2002;16:14–25.
[30] Murphy A. Stress levels and health status of victims of a natural disaster. Res Nurs Health 1984;7:205–15.
[31] Weinrich S, Weinrich M, Hardin S, et al. Effects of psychological distress on blood pressure in adolescents. Holist Nurs Pract 2000;15:57–65.

Nurs Clin N Am 40 (2005) 523–533

NURSING CLINICS
OF NORTH AMERICA

LSEVIER
AUNDERS

Practical Considerations for Providing Pediatric Care in a Mass Casualty Incident

Susan McDaniel Hohenhaus, RN, MA

Pediatric Emergency Department, Duke University, Box 3055, Durham, NC 27710, USA

E mergency preparedness responders have the difficult job of planning for the unknown. Although the extent of illness or injury associated with a mass casualty incident (MCI) in a given community cannot be anticipated fully, some degree of health care planning is possible. Special patient populations have unique needs that can be identified before an incident. If those needs are known, specific plans can be implemented to help reduce the risks those populations may encounter in a disaster.

Children are a special population because of their multiple unique physiological and developmental characteristics that can impede their ability to withstand a major illness or injury (see Table 1). If an entire community is threatened, and the unique needs of children have not been addressed in pre-event plans, they may be overlooked as responders make decisions based on the greater good for the largest number of people. This article outlines problems that have been identified in providing care to children during MCIs and provides considerations for delivering pediatric care.

CHALLENGES IN PROVIDING PEDIATRIC CARE IN DISASTERS
Pre-event planning

Children can be found throughout the community and for a portion of the day tend to be in large groups (eg, day care centers, schools, and sporting events). In the event of a disaster, the number of anticipated child victims will be proportional to their general representation in the overall population. There are exceptions, such as if children are primary targets (eg, 2004 terrorist takeover of a school in Chechnya) or secondary targets (eg, 1995 Oklahoma City bombing) in terrorist events or if a disaster selectively affects where children are grouped.

Injured or ill children who need medical attention often are transported to the nearest community hospitals. Even in nondisasters, most children are seen

E-mail address: susan.hohenhaus@duke.edu

0029-6465/05/$ – see front matter
doi:10.1016/j.cnur.2005.04.014

Table 1
Considerations for the unique pediatric physiology during mass casualty incident

Issue	Physiologic vulnerability	Solution
Exposure to aerosolized chemical	Increased respiratory rate causes increased absorption.	Early recognition and basic airway management
Agents absorbed through skin	Increased body surface area and thinner skin cause increased absorption	Early decontamination recognizing need to prevent hypothermia
Agents causing vomiting and diarrhea	Increase risk of rapid dehydration	Early consideration of vascular access and fluid replacement
Narrow window for recognition and treatment of hypovolemia	Smaller circulating blood volumes	Early consideration of vascular access and fluid/blood replacement
Need for correctly sized equipment and correct medication doses	Requirement for different sized equipment and varying medication doses based on weight	Standardization and organization of pediatric equipment and identification of medications by weight

in nonspecialty centers; therefore, general care practitioners need to anticipate the need to be able to treat large numbers of children during an MCI. According to data from 1997, children and adolescents accounted for 41.2 visits among 100 patients to emergency departments (ED) in the United States [1]. In a survey conducted by the Consumer Product Safety Commission, it was estimated that only 10% of hospitals in the survey had specialized pediatric emergency or critical care facilities, yet 76% of those hospitals admitted children [2]. The American Academy of Pediatrics (AAP) has stated that "community hospitals must have the equipment and skilled personnel to recognize, stabilize, and support the timely transport of pediatric patients to a prearranged definitive care resource" [3]. This view has been supported by multiple organizations [3].

Developing standards for pediatric care

Planners sometimes assume that if a health care institution has the general pieces in place for disaster preparedness, that they have covered the basic needs of all patients. This assumption could prove to be a major disservice for pediatric patients. Children and adolescents do not always fit well into adult-oriented plans.

There have been efforts to introduce standards for pediatric emergency care. In 1991, the 7th World Congress on Emergency and Disaster Medicine created the International Committee on Pediatric Disaster Medicine [4]. The committee was developed to provide assistance to children in any disaster. In 1984, the US Congress approved the Emergency Medical Services for

Children (EMSC) program to expand and improve services for children needing treatment for trauma or critical care. The program is financed by grants to states or schools of medicine and is administered by several federal agencies. In the 1990s, several medical associations developed guidelines for emergency preparedness for pediatric patients. In 1993, the Emergency Nurses Association developed the Emergency Nurses Pediatric Course.

Challenges associated with delivering pediatric care
Defining the pediatric patient
One of the initial challenges that planners and providers encounter is a lack of a consensus on how to define the pediatric population.

Age. Not all professional sources use the same definition of what age constitutes a pediatric patient. The AAP defines childhood from birth to age 21 years, but the American Heart Association (AHA) defines infancy as birth to age 1 year and childhood as 1 to 8 years. Adding to the confusion, health care policies and protocols may switch between the definitions. For example, an emergency medical services (EMS) agency may define a child by the AHA guidelines; the pediatric ED accepts children up to age 16, and the Pediatric Intensive Care Unit (PICU) may accept children to age 13. In the MCI setting, children's ages are difficult to estimate without an accurate historian, such as a parent, teacher, or caregiver [5].

Weight. Emergency medical services and hospital-based providers have used body weight to predict body mass and size of equipment and to calculate drug doses. Unfortunately, accurate weights are difficult to obtain in an MCI.

Error-prone calculations
On-the-spot drug calculations and the use of formulas to determine correct equipment size can be prone to error when the clinician is stressed. In one study involving on-site ED observations made by expert pediatric clinicians, it was noted that staff were confused, uncomfortable, and lacked adherence to pediatric protocols when addressing the resuscitation of a single simulated pediatric patient [6]. There is extensive literature documenting the high rate of errors made when performing drug calculations [7]. Clinicians not only have conflicting definitions of what is a pediatric patient, but resources also vary regarding appropriate medication doses and equipment size.

CONSIDERATIONS FOR PROVIDING PEDIATRIC CARE IN A MASS CASUALTY INCIDENT
Pre-event planning
Recommended guide for care
One system that can be used in any emergency setting is a pediatric emergency measuring tape (Fig. 1). The tape was introduced in the late 1980s and is considered as an accurate and reliable standard for estimating weight in an emergently ill or injured pediatric patient who is younger than 13 years old [8–10].

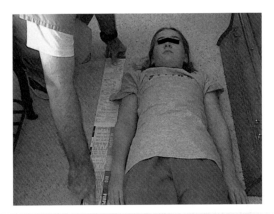

Fig. 1. Demonstration of how to assess child's length using a pediatric measuring tape.

A supine child is placed on a flat surface, and the tape provides for a quick determination of height and estimated weight. The tape assigns a color zone to body length (see Fig. 1), and the color zone that corresponds with the child's length has pre-calculated medication doses for resuscitation drugs and equipment sizes. Emergency care providers have documented that this system has improved their organization and comfort when caring for seriously ill or injured children [11].

Anticipate lack of prehospital triage
During an emergency, it is not uncommon for families and caregivers to take children from the scene to the ED without field intervention. Hospital-based providers will need to recall the unique physiologic vulnerabilities that children have and how children respond differently to injury and illness than adults. According to the AAP Task Force on Terrorism, key pediatric disaster resuscitation issues include:

- Increased vulnerability to aerosolized biological or chemical agents and agents absorbed through the skin
- Agents that produce vomiting or diarrhea increase a child's risk of rapid dehydration.
- Children (because of their smaller circulating blood volumes) have a narrow window for the clinician to recognize and treat profound shock
- Children need appropriately sized equipment and medication dosages.
- Children present special challenges with decontamination efforts.

These factors require a "global size-up" [12,13].

Establish protocols for care
Because it would be nearly impossible to procure expert advice during an actual MCI event, agencies need to develop specific protocols and guidelines ahead of time. Resources, such as an experienced pharmacist or toxicologist can be used to identify pediatric medication and antidote dosing for use in an MCI,

and alternative routes of medication administration. For instance, atropine, pralidoxime (2-PAM chloride) and benzodiazepines are antidotes for nerve agents that usually are given intravenously. If it is not possible or feasible to administer the drugs in this manner during an MCI, they can be administered intramuscularly. Clinicians will need to know doses for both intravenous (IV) and intramuscular (IM) routes and how to reconstitute pralidoxime for IM dosing to avoid a large volume of medication [14]. Reference materials should be stored in an antidote locker with the medications.

Create pediatric antidote kits
Several currently available antidote kits (eg, cyanide) are designed for use in industrial exposure (absorption or ingestion). Typically, most hospitals have one or a few cyanide kits and extra atropine and amyl nitrite available. In the event of an MCI, it is unlikely that there will be enough kits available. Kits also may be an expensive way to store these antidotes.

Organize and store pediatric equipment in one setting
Several items are needed to care for a surge of pediatric patients in an MCI. A designated pediatric storage area could be used to consolidate essential equipment and to help organize the distribution of critical supplies during a crisis.

Anticipate the need for extra personnel
Children lack the cognitive ability to make clear and rational decisions and may not respond to commands or directions. They may react unpredictably, such as show no fear of a dangerous device or substance or become confused and extremely frightened when they are separated from their caregiver. An MCI plan should include additional people who can help comfort children. There may be a need for mental health professionals if children are frightened, anxious, or psychologically traumatized.

Children with special needs may not be able to ambulate or speak. They may have chronic respiratory problems or an altered neurological status, making it difficult to know if the child has an acute or chronic condition. Because caregivers can be separated from children, schools, day care centers and other child-oriented agencies could be encouraged to keep brief medical data cards readily available to be sent with children. In some cases, cards that contain a description of the child's special needs are sent on buses and other transport vehicles and are kept near the driver's seat.

Delivering care during an event
Use pediatric triage systems
A rapid assessment is essential to determine how urgently a child needs care. Several triage models available.

Pediatric Assessment Triangle. The AAP initially developed the Pediatric Assessment Triangle (PAT) (see Table 2) as part of an Emergency Medical Services for Children (EMS-C) federal project, and introduced the concept in

Table 2
Use of the pediatric assessment triangle for possible chemical agent identification

Appearance	Work of breathing	Circulation to skin	Possible chemical agent
Abnormal: seizures, pinpoint pupils	Increased excessive pulmonary secretions	Normal or abnormal	Nerve agent (ie, organophosphate)
Abnormal: normal of large pupils	Respiratory distress or arrest	Flushed	Cyanide
Abnormal: excessive tearing of eyes	Respiratory distress, pulmonary edema	Normal or abnormal	Choking agent (ie, chlorine)

2000. PAT uses visual and auditory clues to develop a first impression of the child, to identify pediatric physiologic instability, and offer a quick (30- to 60-second), standardized approach to triage, resuscitation, treatment, and transport.

The components of the PAT include appearance, work of breathing, and circulation to the skin. The clinician can evaluate a child's oxygenation, ventilation, and cerebral perfusion without using sophisticated tools or instruments. Instead, the child is inspected for work of breathing and signs of skin circulation and auditory sounds of distress.

Work of breathing is evaluated by listening for abnormal airway sounds (eg, gurgling, stridor, or wheezing) and looking for signs of increased breathing effort (ie, abnormal positioning, retractions, or nasal flaring). Combining the assessment for appearance and work of breathing can help determine respiratory distress from respiratory failure or impending respiratory arrest. A rapid assessment of skin circulation for pallor, mottling, and cyanosis can help to determine the adequacy of perfusion of vital organs. An abnormal skin appearance suggests that the child is hypoperfusing. By combining all three components of the PAT, the clinician should be able to determine if the child has a potential physiological abnormality associated with an illness or injury [15]. The child has a less mature blood brain barrier, which makes him or her more susceptible to the neurological effects of chemical agents (Table 1).

The PAT can be used to assess children during any patient encounter. Practice during routine emergency care can help to assure ease and familiarity with the technique, so that it will allow for an increase in critical thinking effort and decision-making capability when there are multiple child victims with varying severities of illness, injury or exposure. A more detailed discussion of the PAT and PEPP is available at www.PEPPsite.com.

START and JumpSTART algorithms. A common algorithm that is used with adult field triage for MCI victims is the Simple Triage and Rapid Treatment (START) [16]. START was developed by the Newport Beach, Calif., Fire and Marine Department and Hoag Hospital. The START program is based on a person's ability to verbally respond and ambulate and their respirations, perfusion, and mental status (RPM). Unfortunately, small children do not all have the ability to verbally communicate or ambulate and tend to have

JumpSTART Pediatric MCI Triage ©

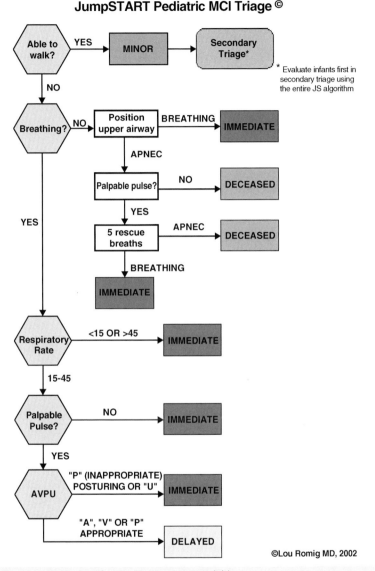

Fig. 2. JumpSTART algorithm (*From* Romig L. Available at: www.jumpstarttriage.com; with permission.)

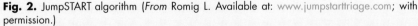

different etiologies for respiratory arrest. Therefore, the START program was modified for use in children and named the JumpSTART program [15] (Fig. 2). JumpSTART can be used for a child who fits within the parameters of the Broselow pediatric emergency tape (Armstrong Medical, Lincolnshire, IL).

In the adult, unless there is clear external airway obstruction or compression of internal airway obstruction from a foreign body, traumatic respiratory failure usually follows circulatory failure or catastrophic head injury. An apneic adult usually has significant cardiac injury (because of hypoperfusion/hypoxia) and is relatively nonsalvageable in the MCI setting.

In children, the opposite is more often true, in that circulatory failure usually follows respiratory failure. Children can become apneic relatively quickly because of mechanical reasons (eg, weak intercostal musculature, inhibition of diaphragmatic excursion, or mechanical airway obstruction) and do not tend to have a prolonged period of hypoxia. There may be a brief period of time in which the child is apneic (or intermittently) but not yet pulseless, because the heart has not experienced prolonged hypoxia. If rescuers clear the airway and start a brief trial of ventilation, the patient may be able to spontaneously breathe. Rescue breathing then will be maintained until further medical assistance is available. This brief trial of ventilation during a period of potential salvageability is a jumpstart for the child, similar to that provided by electrical defibrillation for adults who are pulseless with a cardiac dysrhythmia.

Infants who are developmentally unable to walk should be screened at the initial site (or at the secondary triage site for green patients if carried there by others), using the JumpSTART algorithm. If they satisfy all of the physiologic delayed criteria (ie, fulfill no immediate criteria) and appear to have no significant external injury, infants may be triaged to the minor category.

All children who are able to walk are directed to an area designated for minor injuries, where they will undergo secondary (more involved) triage. At a minimum, secondary triage should consist of RPM.

Special needs children who cannot talk or ambulate should be triaged similar to infants. The initial triage guidelines should be used to assess respiratory, circulatory, or neurological function, and secondary triage can be used to differentiate if the changes are caused by acute or chronic problems. Information about how to implement JumpSTART can be found at: www.jumpstarttriage.com.

When a suspected chemical exposure occurs, the only clues to the type of chemical involved may be the victims' symptoms (Table 2). The PAT triage system allows a rescuer to readily identify significant changes, such as pupil size, excessive tearing, skin signs of irritation, blistering, or chemical burn. Chemical agents tend to affect the work of breathing by changing either the rate (increased or decreased) or amount of pulmonary secretions. Depending on the cause, the patient can have signs of altered skin circulation. Nerve agents (eg, tabun; sarin; soman; cyclosarin; VX; organophosphates) produce symptoms of excessive parasympathetic nervous system stimulation: salivation, lacrimation, urination, defecation, gastrointestinal distress (diarrhea and emesis) (SLUDGE). These symptoms may cause more distress and instability in children, as children tend to become dehydrated more quickly.

Modify emergency interventions to fit the patient and situation
Resuscitation is focused on decontamination, airway control, providing 100% oxygen, supportive care (eg, fluids), and antidote administration. The purpose

of this section is not to review all indicated emergency care, instead it is to highlight the special considerations that should be given to children involved in an MCI.

Decontamination. All children should be considered as potentially contaminated before rescuers attempt to pick them up or hold them. This basic rule will allow rescuers to hold their sympathies in check and avoid becoming a secondary victim. In many cases, decontamination should consist of fresh air and a large volume of low pressure, warm water. The process of decontamination could be more difficult with children who are hesitant to disrobe or go through a shower without a trusted caregiver. Agencies should establish and test policies to determine how best to handle these issues. Child victims will need to be watched for potential hypothermia. Their smaller surface-to-body area ratio and lack of subcutaneous tissue allows for a greater heat loss when they are wet.

Airway management. If large numbers of children are involved in an MCI, rescuers have to be realistic about how they can control airways. Although endotracheal intubation is the standard for critically ill patients, the process is challenging when done in a controlled environment. Simultaneously intubating and successfully maintaining intubation in a large number of children would be even more difficult. As an alternative, care providers can use an oral airway to keep the oropharynx patent and a bag-valve-mask to provide ventilations. This option would be labor-intensive but could be an effective alternative method for large numbers of pediatric patients. Planners would need to plan for additional infant-, child-, and adult-sized airways, bag-valve-masks, and oxygen masks.

Fluid administration. Health care providers should anticipate that gaining and maintaining IV access in a large number of children during an MCI will be problematic. If IV access is not possible, and the child critically needs fluids, providers may consider intraosseous access.

Antidote administration. There are several issues that need to be addressed when considering how to treat children with antidotes. How best to calculate antidote dosage for children involved in an MCI remains unresolved. General care providers should work with pediatric emergency and disaster medicine consultants to explore this and similar issues ahead of an event. Currently, antidotes have not been correlated to the color zones of the Broselow pediatric emergency tape.

The route and indications for antidotes can be different in children compared with adults. Certain antidotes (eg, for cyanide-type poisonings: hydrogen cyanide, cyanogen chloride, or arsenic trihydride) must be given intravenously. If IV access is not feasible when working with large numbers of patients, clinicians should recall that multiple drugs can be given safely by other routes. Some drugs may be given intramuscularly or inhaled by means of the bag-valve-mask device. Many chemical agents can induce vomiting and diarrhea; therefore oral or rectal medications should not be considered as alternate routes for emergency treatment.

Using prepackaged medications can present a special challenge if the products are not the correct dose for children. Henretig and colleagues [17] studied the feasibility of having rescuers dressed in full personal protective equipment manipulate the prefilled medication autoinjectors found in a prepackaged adult Mark 1 kit. The subjects were instructed to discharge the medications into small sterile vials, then aspirate the desired dose (ie, on 1 mg/kg basis) for administration to small children. The investigators observed that the fully garbed subjects could successfully inject the antidotes from the autoinjectors into the vials and access a 1 mg/kg dose with little difficulty in dexterity or learning curve. The authors concluded that the potential reuse of prepackaged antidote autoinjectors might provide a way to deliver medications to children in the event of a biochemical mass casualty incident.

In an MCI, clinicians may have to use different guidelines for determining when to use antidotes in children. For some patients, the most likely route of large-scale chemical exposure would be by inhalation (eg, cyanide). If after patients are removed from the environment, they continue to breathe, have no significant worsening of symptoms, survive until EMS arrives or they are transported to the hospital, they might survive without an antidote. Theoretically, patients who are breathing should continue to breathe and steadily improve. This assumption is valid if inhalation was the only route of exposure. If cyanide was aerosolized and primarily inhaled by adults, children who are lower to the ground might continue to absorb droplets cutaneously from the air and therefore need antidotes.

Not all antidotes have been used in children; therefore, the literature may be lacking in pediatric indications or dosages. For example, the nitrogen mustards are treated with British Anti Lewisite (BAL). There is little reported experience using BAL with children.

SUMMARY

Children involved in an MCI can be primary or secondary victims. Health care providers need to remember that children have unique vulnerabilities to injuries and illnesses that may be caused by MCIs, particularly in the case of chemical exposure. Pediatric victims most likely will be seen in community centers, and providers need to be prepared to address their vulnerabilities. Preparing for a surge in pediatric patients, using predetermined guides for calculating interventions, and modifying care during an MCI are critical and practical considerations that can improve the outcome for children. Child advocates must encourage local, state, regional, and federal agencies to incorporate policies, procedures, and protocols that are practical and universal and that reduce error by simplifying the process.

References

[1] Weiss HB, Mathers LJ, Forjuoh SN, et al. Child and adolescent emergency department visit data book. Pittsburgh (PA): Center for Violence and Injury Control, Allegheny University of the Health Sciences; 1997.

[2] Athey J, Dean JS, Ball J, et al. Ability of hospitals to care for pediatric emergency patients. Pediatr Emerg Care 2001;17:170–4.

[3] American Academy of Pediatrics Committee on Pediatric Emergency Medicine. Guidelines for pediatric emergency care facilities. Pediatrics 1995;13(2):526–37.

[4] Roshal LM. Pediatric disasters. Available at: http://pdm.medicine.wisc.edu/roshal1.htm. Accessed February 28, 2005.

[5] Harris M, Patterson J, Morse J. Doctors, nurses and parents are equally poor at estimating pediatric weights. Pediatr Emerg Care 1999;15(1):17–8.

[6] Hohenhaus S. Is this a drill? Improving pediatric emergency preparedness in North Carolina's emergency departments. J Emerg Nurs 2001;27(6):568–70.

[7] Selbst S, Fein J, Osterhoudt K, et al. Medication errors in a pediatric emergency department. Pediatr Emerg Care 1999;15(1):1–4.

[8] Lubitz DS, Seidel JS, Chameides L, et al. A rapid method for estimating weight and resuscitation drug dosages from length in a pediatric group. Ann Emerg Med 1988; 17:576–81.

[9] Luten RC, Wears RL, Broselow J, et al. Length based endotracheal tube and emergency equipment in pediatrics. Ann Emerg Med 1992;21:900–4.

[10] Luten RC. Pediatric resuscitation chart and equipment shelf: aids to mastery of age related problems. J Emerg Med 1986;4:9–14.

[11] Grem C. One emergency department's system for improved pediatric codes. J Emerg Nurs 1994;20:118–21.

[12] Romig L. PREP for peds-patient physiology, rescuer responses, equipment, protocols and size up and approach tips for pediatric calls. JEMS 2001;26(5):24–33.

[13] Howard PK. Pediatric education for prehospital professionals. J Emerg Nurs 2000; 26(5):481–2.

[14] Taketomo CK, Hodding JS, Kraus DM. Pediatric dosage handbook. 9th edition. Hudson (OH): Lexi-Comp, Incorporated; 2002.

[15] Romig L. Pediatric triage. A system to JumpSTART your triage of young patients at MCIs. JEMS 2002;52(8):60–3.

[16] Risavi BL, Salen PN, Heller MB, et al. A two-hour intervention using START improves prehospital triage of mass casualty incidents. Prehosp Emerg Care 2001;5(2):197–9.

[17] Henretig FM, Mechem C, Jew R. Potential use of autoinjector-packaged antidotes for treatment of pediatric nerve agent toxicity. Ann Emerg Med 2002;40(4):405–8.

Nurs Clin N Am 40 (2005) 535–550

NURSING CLINICS
OF NORTH AMERICA

Disaster Care: Psychological Considerations

Ann M. Mitchell, PhD, RN[a],*, Teresa J. Sakraida, DNSc, RN[a], Kirstyn K. Zalice, MSN, CRNP[b]

[a]University of Pittsburgh School of Nursing, 415 Victoria Building, Pittsburgh, PA 15261, USA
[b]Robert Morris University, School of Nursing and Allied Health, 6001 University Boulevard, Moon Township, PA 15108, USA

Disasters are tragic events that disrupt the normal functioning of a community [1] and overwhelm personal and community resources. The events can be caused by natural forces (ie, caused by environmental changes) or human-made (eg, industrial explosions, hazardous spills, nuclear release, or intentional acts). Whatever the etiology, disasters cause loss of physical property and emotional distress. A sudden event that precipitates fear of injury or loss of life can be described as an emotionally traumatic event because lives are changed (of the victims, survivors, family members, neighbors, and helpers). The people who experience or simply witness traumatic events can be affected emotionally and develop a range of physical and emotional responses, which in turn can produce psychological, social, and physiological dysfunction.

The challenge for health care providers is to recognize the range of emotions and to be able to identify when professional help is indicated. This article provides an overview of the human stress response and describes sources of stress that follow disasters, acute stress disorder (ASD), post-traumatic stress disorder (PTSD), and interventions and resources used to care for victims after disasters.

HUMAN STRESS RESPONSE

Hans Selye described stress as the nonspecific response of the body to any type of demand, and factors that produce stress are referred to as stressors, which can be acute or chronic [2]. Psychoneuroimmunology evaluates how the neuroendocrine system responds to stress and the physiological changes that follow. Acute stressors (eg, a decreased oxygen supply, pain, acute infections, noise, malnutrition, heat, cold, and trauma) involve physiological demands or emotional reactions (eg, anxiety, fear, depression, anger, and excitement) [3].

*Corresponding author. E-mail address: ammi@pitt.edu (A.M. Mitchell).

0029-6465/05/$ – see front matter
doi:10.1016/j.cnur.2005.04.006

Chronic physiological stressors may include: obesity, prolonged drug use, numerous chronic diseases, and some medical treatments [4]. How individuals ultimately respond to acute or chronic stressors depends upon their personality, their perception of the threat, and their current and past coping skills. When stressors are overwhelming, homeostasis is disturbed, and stress-related symptoms may develop (Table 1).

SOURCES OF STRESS
Disasters and terrorist attacks expose innumerable people to scenes of death, destruction, or human loss. An individual who has been directly exposed to, experienced, witnessed, or confronted with death (actual or threatened) or serious injury can respond with intense fear, helplessness, or horror [5]. Physical integrity is threatened, and the person may be at a high risk for emotional trauma. Additionally, people can be victimized by the secondary effects of a disaster, such as mass media coverage, the need for temporary relocation, and financial problems that may inflict an additive burden onto the primary or direct effects of loss. The degree of change required for adjustment will affect the individual's appraisal and meaning of the loss, which may lead to perceptions of stress [6]. People also may have increased uncertainty about the future and with a terrorist attack, a greater sense of insecurity that stems from discordant world–state relations.

RESPONSES TO STRESS
A study [7] conducted within 2 months after the collapse of the World Trade Center in 2001 assessed the prevalence of depression and PTSD among the residents of Manhattan. Among the 1008 adults interviewed, 9.7% reported

Table 1
Common symptoms and reactions of disaster survivors

Affective	Behavioral	Cognitive	Physical
Depression, sadness, and/or mood swings	Difficulty falling or staying asleep	Confusion and/or disorientation	Tiredness, fatigue, or exhaustion
Irritability and/or angry outbursts	Crying easily and tearfulness	Recurrent dreams and/or nightmares	Gastrointestinal distress
Fear, anxiety, and/or verbalized distress	Avoiding reminders of the event	Preoccupation with trauma	Increased or decreased appetite
Despair, hopelessness, and/or helplessness	Hyperactivity or hypoactivity	Difficulty concentrating	Numerous somatic complaints
Self-doubt, guilt, and/or blame	Increased conflicts with others	Questioning spiritual beliefs	Exacerbation of prior health problems

Adapted from DeWolfe DJ. Training manual for mental health and human service workers in major disasters. (ADM Publication No. 90-538). Washington DC: US Department of Human Services. Plum KC. Understanding the psychosocial impact of disasters. In: Veenema TG, editor. Disaster and emergency preparedness for chemical, biological, radiological terrorism and other hazards. New York: Springer Publishing; 2003:63–81.

symptoms consistent with depression, and 7.5% reported symptoms consistent with PTSD. The number of adults with symptoms of PTSD increased to 20% for those residents living closest to the World Trade Center. The greatest predictor of depression was suffering personal losses as a result of the attacks. Experiences that involved direct exposure to the attacks were the greatest predictors of PTSD symptoms.

Intentional acts that use biological and chemical weaponry are intended to introduce fear, confusion, and greater uncertainty into everyday life [8]. Common psychological reactions to bioterrorism include: (1) horror or panic; (2) fear of invisible agents or fear of contagion; (3) anger at terrorists, the government or both; (4) scapegoating or loss of faith in social institutions; and (5) paranoia, social isolation, or demoralization [9].

EMOTIONAL RECOVERY AND PSYCHIATRIC SEQUELAE

Various efforts have been used to help classify phases of a disaster and mitigating factors that affect emotions [6,10,11]. The range of possible emotional responses suggests that people use several variables to recover. Early models of recovery did not provide for an evaluation of mediating processes or their role in recovery. To fill this theoretical void, Murphy [6] proposed an explanatory model that addressed the person's role in recovery and identified three broad dimensions that influence recovery. These dimensions are: the occurrence of the event and its significance to the individual, the individual's personal attributes, and mediating processes.

Although there are multiple factors that can affect how a person responds, the perception of numerous losses generally has a negative impact and may be related inversely to disaster recovery. Environmental and social mediating factors, such as perceived social support, social networks, and community resources, also can affect a person's response to a disaster. Murphy [6] concludes that these variables act directly or indirectly on recovery from disasters.

Austin and Godleski [12] reported that slightly more than half (up to 60%) of individuals exposed to a disaster will develop psychiatric symptoms immediately after the event. This number drops to 41% by 10 weeks and to 22% by 1 year. When loss of life and physical injury following a disaster is minimal, psychiatric sequelae may be relatively low. Conversely, when an event produces an immediate overwhelming number of deaths and high levels of symptoms, then the presence of long-term psychiatric disorders may be quite high [13].

Data on long-term emotional recovery from disasters remain inconsistent. Whereas incidents of extreme psychopathologies are rare, more information about emotional disturbances and adaptive coping responses is needed [14,15]. Baseline data show that a certain portion of the population is at risk for developing maladaptive responses. Epidemiological surveys of large groups of the general public determined that lifetime exposure to traumatic events may be as high as 73.6% for men and 64.8% for women [16]. Community-based studies show the prevalence of developing PTSD for any person during his or her lifetime ranges from 1% to 14% for all [5] to 5% of men and 10% to 12% of women [17]. This figure jumps from 3% to 58% for at-risk individuals [5].

Not every person is affected or responds the same way after a traumatic event. Individuals can express varying degrees of distress and different signs of recovery. Although most emotionally traumatized survivors will recover without the need for external intervention [14], some individuals experience intense stress and will have a greater risk of developing maladaptive responses or psychiatric comorbidities. As time passes, and the immediate threat diminishes, victims may begin to manifest other psychological responses that will need assessment and possibly need intervention. Emotional responses that can be expected include depression, anxiety, complicated bereavement reactions, substance use, physical health problems, functional disabilities, ASD, and PTSD. Assessment is important to differentiate the symptoms of ASD from PTSD and entails understanding the typical characteristics of each disorder (Table 2).

Acute stress disorder

Persons closest to the emotionally traumatic event are at the greatest risk for developing ASD. Characteristics of ASD are the development of certain signs and symptoms (ie, anxiety or disassociation) and the timing of the symptoms (ie, occurring within 1 month after the trauma and lasting a minimum of 2 days and a maximum of 4 weeks) [5].

In considering a diagnosis of ASD, two features must be present. First, the person must have experienced, witnessed, or have been confronted with an event or events that involved actual or threatened death, or serious injury, or a threat to the physical integrity of self or others. Additionally, the person's response must have involved intense fear, helplessness, or horror [5]. Furthermore, the individual must have three or more dissociative symptoms (see Box 1). The presence of a predisposing condition, such as past psychological trauma, also may increase the likelihood of this disorder. If symptoms persist longer than 4 weeks post-trauma, a diagnosis of PTSD should be considered. Because the likelihood of developing PTSD is increased for those having ASD, the assessment of individuals for the presence of ASD is a key factor in identifying those at risk of developing future complications.

Post-traumatic stress disorder

Post-traumatic stress disorder is a response to witnessing a traumatic event that involves interpersonal violence, grotesque sensory images, or some natural disaster. As with ASD, the individual will have been confronted with an event or events that involved actual or threatened death or serious injury, and the person's responses will have involved intense fear, helplessness, or horror. Individuals also experience impairment in social, occupational, or other functioning [5].

Table 2
Comparison of acute stress and post-traumatic stress disorders

The person (1) experienced, witnessed, or was confronted with an event that involved actual or threatened death to self or others, and 2) responded with fear, helplessness, or horror.

Acute stress disorder (ASD)	Post-traumatic stress disorder (PTSD)
Lasts from 2 days to 4 weeks and occurs within 4 weeks of the traumatic/disaster event	Duration more than 1 month and may be acute, chronic, or delayed
Three or more dissociative symptoms: ■ Numbness and/or detachment ■ Reduced awareness of surroundings ■ Derealization and/or depersonalization ■ Amnesia or memory loss	Dissociative symptoms are not part of the Diagnostic and Statistical Manual of Mental Disorders, Fourth Edition, Test Revision criteria for PTSD.
The event is re-experienced in at least one of the following ways: ■ Distressing dreams or images ■ A sense of reliving the event ■ Flashbacks, illusions	The event is re-experienced in one or more of the following ways: ■ Recurrent and intrusive distressing recollections of the traumatic event ■ Recurrent distressing dreams or nightmares ■ Feeling as if the event were recurring, through flashbacks, illusions, hallucinations ■ Psychological distress at exposure to internal or external cues ■ Physiological reactivity
Marked avoidance of stimuli that arouse memories or recollections of the trauma including: ■ People and places ■ Activities and conversations ■ Thoughts and feelings	Persistent avoidance of stimuli associated with the trauma by three or more of the following: ■ Isolation from family/friends ■ Feelings of numbness ■ Excessive fatigue ■ Moodiness ■ Restricted range of affect ■ Sense of foreshortened future
Marked symptoms of increased arousal or anxiety including: ■ Difficulty falling or staying asleep ■ Irritability or outbursts of anger ■ Difficulty concentrating ■ Motor restlessness	Persistent symptoms of increased arousal of two or more of the following: ■ Restlessness ■ Sleep disturbance ■ Irritability or angry outbursts ■ Startle reactions ■ Suspiciousness ■ Hypervigilance

Adapted from American Psychiatric Association. Diagnostic and statistical manual of mental disorders. 4th edition. Washington (DC): American Psychiatric Association; 1994.

Post-traumatic stress disorder is recognized by means of a diagnostic cluster of symptoms (see Box 2 for the three symptom clusters associated with PTSD). Individuals vividly re-experience or relive the event and may have flashbacks that generally last only a few seconds. They demonstrate avoidance behaviors, which are efforts to ignore or suppress thoughts or feelings about the incident, and thirdly, they may complain of symptoms of increased physiological arousal

Box 1: Assessment of acute stress disorder dissociative symptom cluster

To assess for detachment symptoms the following questions might be asked:

- Have you recently noticed a sense of numbness or detachment?
- Are you feeling emotionally numb?

To assess for awareness of surrounding symptoms the following questions might be asked:

- Are you noticing that you are having difficulty staying focused or being aware of your surroundings?
- Do you feel as if you are in a daze?

To assess for symptoms of derealization and depersonalization symptoms the following questions might be asked:

- Have you been feeling as if the environment is unreal or strange in any way?
- Have you been feeling unreal, strange, or unfamiliar with yourself?
- Do you feel as if you are outside of your body in any way?

To assess for dissociative symptoms the following questions might be asked:

- Do you have periods of memory loss?
- Are you having difficulty recalling important aspects of the disaster/ traumatic event?

Adapted from American Psychiatric Association. Diagnostic and statistical manual of mental disorders. 4th edition. Washington (DC): American Psychiatric Association; 1994.

[5]. The diagnosis of PTSD requires that symptoms be present for at least 1 month after the event. It is considered to be acute if the duration of symptoms is less than 3 months and chronic if the symptoms persist beyond 3 months. PTSD can be considered delayed-onset if the symptoms do not appear until after 6 months following the traumatic event [5].

Certain individuals are at an increased risk for PTSD, such as women and anyone lacking social support, experiencing chronic fear and feelings of helplessness, lacking strong political or religious affiliation, having an all-or-nothing view of events, and a prior history of psychiatric illness [18,19]. Victims of PTSD have a high incidence of comorbid conditions, including major depression, panic disorder, generalized anxiety disorder, and substance abuse [20]. Two studies found that a lifetime history of at least one other psychiatric disorder was present in 88.3% of men with lifetime PTSD and 79% of the women with lifetime PTSD [20,21]. Somatization disorder (ie, persons presenting with numerous physical complaints, seeking treatment, and interfering with functioning) frequently has been noted with PTSD. One study [21] found somatization disorder was present 90 times more frequently in those with PTSD than in persons without it. This suggests an important connection between PTSD and numerous physical complaints [21,22].

Box 2: Assessment of post-traumatic stress disorder three symptom clusters

To assess for re-experiencing symptoms, the following questions might be asked:

- Are you troubled by recurrent thoughts or images of the traumatic event?
- Have you had recurrent nightmares about the event?
- Are you having any periods in which you felt as if the event was reoccurring?
- Have you had any flashbacks of the event?
- Have you experienced any hallucinations?
- Are you experiencing psychological distress?
- Have you noticed any physical symptoms such as sweating, increased heart rate, shortness of breath, or shakiness?

To assess for avoidance and/or numbing symptoms, the following questions might be asked:

- Are you noticing that you are trying to avoid thinking or talking about the traumatic event?
- Are you having difficulty remembering any aspects of the event?
- Have you experienced a decrease or lack of interest in activities that were once enjoyable for you?
- Have you had difficulty socializing and enjoying being around people?
- Do you feel detached from people around you?
- Have you had difficulties expressing your feelings?
- Do you feel emotionally numb?
- Do you feel as if your future is shortened since the event?
- Do you feel hopeless about the future?

To assess for symptoms of increased arousal, the following questions might be asked:

- Have you had any difficulty with falling asleep or staying asleep since the traumatic event?
- Tell me how your mood has been affected by the event.
- Have you noticed an increase in anger or irritability since the event?
- Have you had problems with your concentration?
- Do you notice that you are easily distracted or preoccupied by thoughts of the event?
- Do you find that you are startled easily when something reminds you of the event?

Adapted from Mitchell AM, Kameg K, Sakraida TJ. Post-traumatic stress: clinical implications. *Disaster Manag Response* 2003;1:14–8.

American Psychiatric Association. Diagnostic and statistical manual of mental disorders. 4th edition. Washington: American Psychiatric Association; 1994.

EMOTIONAL CARE FOR DISASTER VICTIMS

Crisis intervention

Most individuals who experience a disaster or traumatic event will recover without intervention. Health care professionals who see people after a disaster should include preparing them and the bereaved for what lies ahead and identifying individuals and families who are in need of additional follow-up care and referrals. Crisis intervention remains the mainstay of disaster management and can be initiated by disaster care providers who actively listen to survivors and assist in problem-solving [18]. Rescuers can ask survivors to describe their problems and current level of functioning, their adaptive coping skills, and what personal, community, and professional resources are available. Rescuers then can help support survivors and others as they develop and implement a sound and workable plan.

Additional steps that can be taken to reduce psychological harm include: the prevention of retraumatization, the prevention of new victimization, and the prevention of medicalizing normal distress reactions [23,24]. Furthermore, social support networks may provide an important resource for coping with the aftermath of disasters and may mitigate the adverse effects of disaster trauma. Mobilizing families, friends, neighbors, and coworkers may be helpful, although difficult, because of associated disruptions following a particular event. Telephone hotlines can be set up; community support groups can be formed, and creative ways to assist with needed material goods for those affected can be coordinated. These efforts may be helpful with providing some means of comfort and emotional strength. Table 3 lists Web resources that offer information on disaster care.

Focused assessment

Nurses, emergency medical personnel, and health care professionals who work with traumatized persons need to respond to victims with empathy while performing a thorough focused assessment for ASD and PTSD. Because the symptoms of ASD and PTSD are often similar to those seen in anxiety, depressive, and other disorders, individuals should be asked specifically if they have been exposed to a traumatic event. If there is a positive history, the timing in seeking health care also should be noted, as ASD symptoms tend to be time-limited.

Clients with suspected stress disorders should be educated about significant symptoms and helped with enhanced coping and treatment options. The National Institute of Mental Health (NIMH) coordinated a workshop [25] to reach a consensus on best practices for victims and survivors of mass violence (see Box 3). Focused questioning also can be used by multi-disciplinary team members to identify comorbid diagnoses. Boxes 1 and 2 show examples of questions to pose during a focused assessment. Accurate assessments will assist with the prompt identification of individuals with ASD or PTSD and lead to timely and precise treatment by the multi-disciplinary team.

Individuals experiencing traumatic events also may have a risk of suicide. Therefore, individuals should be asked about current suicidal thoughts,

Table 3	
Web resources	
Website	Resource
Federal Emergency Management Agency http://www.fema.gov	Strategic plan with agency goals/objectives Disaster preparedness information
US Department of Health and Human Services, Office of Public Health Emergency Preparedness http://www.ndms.dhhs.gov/index.html	National Disaster Medical System disaster teams
Disaster Relief–Worldwide Disaster Aid and Information http://www.disasterrelief.org	Worldwide disaster information and services
American Hospital Association http://www.hospitalconnect.com/aha/key_issues/disaster_readiness/resources/HospitalReady.html	Hospital readiness, response, and recovery resources
American Nurses Association http://nursingworld.org/ojin/	See Online Journal of Nursing Issues. Click on journal topics and select aftermath of September 11, 2001 (Vol. 7, Issue 3; 2002)
American Psychological Association http://www.apa.org/topics/topic_trauma.html	Information about disaster mental health, fostering resiliency, and warning signs of trauma-related stress
American Red Cross http://www.redcross.org/services/disaster	Disaster preparedness and disaster relief services
Center for Disease Control and Prevention http://www.bt.cdc.gov/	Agents, diseases and other threats (chemical and radiation); Disaster preparedness

presence of plan and intent, or history of previous suicide attempts. The history is not considered to be complete until it also includes an in-depth assessment of drug and alcohol use.

Psychological therapies

There are various types of psychological interventions available for clients with stress disorders. Psychological therapies appear to be more effective for treating ASD and PTSD than psychotropic medications alone [26].

Behavioral therapy

Behavioral therapy often is used to manage the fear experienced by victims and to relieve anxiety [20,27]. Individuals are educated to control the anxiety symptoms by concentrating on breathing exercises and progressive muscle relaxation. Patients can be taught to manage the feared stimulus with

Box 3: Key components of early intervention

Provision for basic needs

• Provide food, shelter, security, and basic first aid
• Assess for ongoing threats
• Orient survivors to available services

Provision for psychological first aid

• Protect survivors from further harm
• Keep families together
• Mobilize services for those most distressed

Provide a needs assessment

• Assess status of individuals, groups, populations, and institutions
• Determine how well needs are being met
• Determine what additional services are needed immediately

Monitor the rescue and recovery environment

• Monitor past and ongoing threats
• Monitor services that are being provided
• Monitor media coverage

Provide for outreach and information dissemination

• Offer information and education as needed
• Utilize established community structures and communication systems
• Conduct media interviews

Foster resilience and recovery

• Provide education on stress responses and normal versus abnormal functioning
• Offer family and group interventions and foster natural social supports
• Provide education on coping skills training and adaptive versus maladaptive coping

Provisions for triage

• Conduct clinical assessments using reliable and valid methods
• Identify vulnerable and high-risk individuals
• Provide emergency hospitalization as necessary

Provide for treatment

• Refer individuals for follow-up care, including pharmacotherapy as needed
• Provide individual, family, and group psychotherapy
• Provide for short and/or long-term hospitalization as necessary

Adapted from National Institute of Mental Health (2002). Mental health and mass violence: evidence-based early psychological intervention for victims/survivors of mass violence: a workshop to reach consensus on best practices. Washington (DC), US Government Printing Office, NIH Publication #02-5138.

Adshead G. Psychological therapies for post-traumatic stress disorder. Br J Psychiatry 2000;177: 144–8.

systematic desensitization. This process involves exposing the person to the feared stimulus/situation for short periods of time to achieve habituation while the individual is in a relaxed state. Over time, the person experiences less anxiety to increased exposures of the feared stimulus/situation.

Cognitive strategies

Cognitive strategies include a form of therapy based on the assumption that an individual's behavior is dependent upon how he or she views the world [20,27]. Patients are assisted in identifying automatic, negative, anxiety-arousing thoughts and replacing those thoughts with supportive and calming self-talk. Cognitive therapy can be combined with behavioral therapy.

Eye movement desensitization and reprocessing

Eye movement desensitization and reprocessing (EMDR) is a controversial form of therapy that has been identified as being effective in treating PTSD. Developed by Shapiro [28], EMDR is designed to facilitate cognitive changes and decrease anxiety. During EMDR, the therapist induces rapid, rhythmic lateral eye movements while the person expresses aversive memories. The individual is asked to bring negative emotions, memories, and cognitions associated with a trauma to the forefront of his/her mind and to restructure negative thoughts into more functional cognitions [28]. There is, however, no evidence that EMDR is a treatment of choice over other approaches [25].

Psychological debriefing

Critical incident stress debriefing (CISD) is one of the most common forms of psychological debriefing, but this is coming under more scrutiny. CISD [23,29] uses some techniques that are common to counseling, but it is not psychotherapy, nor a substitute for psychotherapy. It is primarily a psycho–educational process that allows for the ventilation and expression of thoughts and feelings associated with a traumatic event. It provides people with the opportunity to become educated about the normal stress response and to learn about adaptive coping strategies. The debriefing process allows participants to verbalize their distress and formulate appropriate concepts about the trauma before false interpretations of the experience become fixed. The intended goals of the psychological debriefing process are to mitigate the impact of a traumatic event and to accelerate the recovery process in people who are experiencing normal stress reactions to abnormal traumatic events [23,29].

Studies of psychological debriefings, including CISD, have produced mixed results. CISD was not designed to be a stand-alone intervention but rather as one part of a broader critical incident stress management (CISM) program. CISM is a multi-component intervention that involves being prepared for a crisis, using precrisis education and training, and finding appropriate follow-up or referral sources when necessary. Everly and Boyle [30], however, conducted a meta-analysis of studies that used CISD as a one-time intervention outside of the CISM multi-component intervention. Their analysis demon-strated a high degree of efficacy when CISD was implemented in a restrictive manual-driven protocol. Only five studies, however, were included in their meta-analysis, with an aggregated total of 341 subjects.

Several meta-analyses [31,32] failed to demonstrate the efficacy of CISD as a single-session, individual-focused, intervention. Both of these meta-analyses involved randomized controlled trials (RCTs) with adequate, although small sample sizes (ie, because of exclusion criteria). Some of these studies also included other kinds of interventions along with the CISD intervention. In addition, there were variations in how the specific CISD intervention was administered.

These meta-analyses identified the importance of avoiding numerous methodological pitfalls commonly found during the review of the current studies. They suggest that future research should clarify the intervention model and provide for an assessment procedure to measure intervention effectiveness [30–34]. The direction of future research to evaluate applications and protocols of CISD also should include designing well-controlled research studies directed toward overcoming the limitations of the past. In addition, there are important CISD variables that remain to be examined. These variables include: appropriate procedures, specific populations, delineation of critical incidents, clearly defined time spans between incident and debriefing, follow-up evaluations, and specifying the number and type of health care professionals involved [35–37].

There is limited evidence that psychological interventions used in the acute post-trauma phase are effective in preventing PTSD. Clinicians should be aware that previously traumatized clients may react in a variety of ways. Some patients may experience a reawakening of repressed traumatic experiences that inevitably may create further problems for recovery. Other clients may find that acute psychological preventative interventions may provide opportunities for working through prior traumas. At present, the effectiveness of psychological debriefings in reducing the psychological distress often associated with traumatic events remains unknown.

Richards [35] reported on a prospective field trial comparing two post-trauma interventions following armed robberies. CISD was implemented as a stand-alone group intervention and compared with an integrated CISM protocol. Psychological morbidity was measured using two post-traumatic stress symptom questionnaires and a general health measure. Psychological morbidity was equivalent in the two groups at 3 days and 1 month after the raid. The CISM group, however, had significantly less post-trauma morbidity 3 to 12 months after the raid, compared with the CISD stand-alone intervention. This is perhaps the first study supplying evidence for the efficacy of crisis interventions post-trauma when they are delivered within the integrated CISM protocol.

The literature continues to support important considerations for practice. Any acute preventative intervention must be linked to follow-up services, such as those described in the wider context of CISM [23,29]. Implications for practice include:

- Implementing the CISD intervention as a group-focused debriefing in the context of the more comprehensive CISM protocol

- Ensuring the adequate training of personnel through formal in-service educational programs
- Providing a measure for the objective assessment of its effectiveness
- Providing for follow-up contact to assess for ASD, PTSD, or other comorbid psychological sequelae

Furthermore, participation in a CISD intervention should not be mandatory, and potential participants should receive adequate psychological assessments [36,37].

Litz and colleagues [36] also have outlined approaches that are empirically supported for individuals exposed to trauma. They recommend supporting the individual to achieve natural resolution by using current personal and natural support systems. If resolution does not occur, their stepped approach involves providing early assessments (at about 1 week) with nonintrusive psychological measures and providing, for those individuals who require professional intervention, a short-term cognitive behavioral therapy (CBT) program (beginning at 4 to 6 weeks) after the traumatic event. They suggest caution against the early provision of CBT as a solution for all post-traumatic symptomatology, however, because of participant dropout rates, and concerns of suitability for early exposure therapy for some individuals [36].

Critical incident stress debriefing continues to be valued by clinicians because of its perceived efficacy. Although CISD may not prevent psychopathology, it may be useful to facilitate screening for individuals who may be at risk. Additionally, it can help disseminate education and referral information and assist in maintaining morale [37]. Preventing PTSD is only one objective of psychological debriefings. Other aims include ameliorating distress and identifying and referring individuals who may be at risk for developing chronic problems. The best evidence for efficacy of clinical intervention is through cumulative empirical findings; however, reports of satisfaction and perceived helpfulness by participants might be sufficient reasons to continue to offer debriefings within the CISM context. Debriefings also provide adequate follow-up assessments and referrals. Richards [35] and Litz and colleagues [36] state that it is premature to cease offering debriefings and call for the study of CISM in empirically rigorous, randomized controlled trials.

MEDICATION MANAGEMENT

Although psychotherapy is seen as the cornerstone of treatment, there remains a place for pharmacotherapy for treating ASD and PTSD. The intensity of client symptoms is sometimes so severe that effective therapy is difficult without the use of medications. Katz and colleagues [38] hypothesize that patients with ASD or PTSD experience a massive uptake of norepinephrine (NE) from the synaptic space, which then overwhelms NE production capabilities, resulting in a depletion of synaptic NE. Tricyclic antidepressants (TCAs), particularly amitriptyline, block the reuptake of NE and serotonin and have been shown to be effective for treating PTSD [39]. Unfortunately, TCAs have a tendency to produce adverse effects, primarily through cholinergic, alpha–adrenergic, and histaminergic blockade.

Other researchers hypothesize that patients with ASD and PTSD have problems with the serotonergic system, and this has led to the use of selective serotonin reuptake inhibitors (SSRIs) for treating PTSD [39]. A meta-analysis of randomized controlled trials using SSRIs for treating PTSD found that SSRIs appear to be useful in treating a range of PTSD symptoms [39]. SSRIs are effective in treating comorbid conditions and have a more favorable adverse effect profile than the TCAs. Therefore, they are considered first-line medications for treating PTSD [39]. Common adverse effects of SSRIs include insomnia, hypersomnia, nausea, diarrhea, constipation, increased anxiety, and sexual dysfunction [40]. When first initiating an SSRI in clients with comorbid anxiety disorders, such as generalized anxiety disorder or panic disorder, the short-term use of a benzodiazepine may be useful to help minimize anxiety [41]. Benzodiazepines with longer half-lives such as clonazepam or lorazepam are less likely to produce tolerance and dependence, but they should be used only for a limited time. Double-blind placebo-controlled studies have failed to support a role for using benzodiazepines alone for treating PTSD [42].

SUMMARY

The management of psychological and emotional outcomes following a disaster or trauma begins with a well-developed plan to decrease the adverse impact of the event on the affective, behavioral, and cognitive capacities of the individual, family, and group. From a multi-disciplinary perspective, it is vital that health care professionals become well-versed in mental health treatment protocols essential to trauma and disaster care. Involvement of psychiatric nurse practitioners and clinical nurse specialists should begin with the early development of comprehensive agency and community disaster plans. It is then that appropriate preparedness, mitigation, response, rescue, recovery, and evaluation processes best can be addressed.

References
[1] Veenema TG. Essentials of disaster planning. In: Veenema TG, editor. Disaster and emergency preparedness for chemical, biological, radiological terrorism and other hazards. New York: Springer Publishing; 2003. p. 3–29.
[2] Selye H. Stress without distress. New York: Signet; 1974.
[3] Agarwal SK, Marshall JD. Stress effects on immunity and its application to clinical immunology. Clin Exp Allergy 2001;31:25–31.
[4] McCance KL, Huether SE. Pathophysiology: the biologic basis for disease in adults and children. St. Louis (MO): Mosby; 1998.
[5] American Psychiatric Association. Diagnostic and statistical manual of mental disorders. 4th edition. Washington (DC): American Psychiatric Association; 1994.
[6] Murphy SA. An explanatory model of recovery from disaster loss. Res in Nurs Health 1989;12:67–76.

[7] Galea S, Ahern J, Resnick H, et al. Psychological sequelae of the September 11, terrorist attacks in New York City. N Engl J Med 2002;346:982–7.

[8] Wessly S, Hyams KC, Bartholomew R. Psychological implications of chemical and biological weapons. BMJ 2001;323:878–9.

[9] Holloway HC, Norwood AE, Fullerton CS, et al. The threat of biological weapons: Prophylaxis and mitigation of psychological and social consequences. JAMA 2002; 278:425–7.

[10] Powell J, Rayner J. Progress notes: disaster investigation, July 1, 1951–June 30, 1952. Englewood (MD): Army Chemical Corps Medical Laboratories; 1952.

[11] Berren M, Biegel A, Ghertner S, et al. A typology for the classification of disasters: implications for intervention. Community Mental Health Journal 1980;16:103–11.

[12] Austin LS, Godleski LS. Therapeutic approaches for survivors of suicide. Psychiatr Clin North Am 1999;22:897–910.

[13] Plum KC. Understanding the psychosocial impact of disasters. In: Veenema TG, editor. Disaster and emergency preparedness for chemical, biological, and radiological terrorism and other hazards. New York: Springer Publishing; 2003. p. 63–81.

[14] Bisson JI, Kitchiner NJ. Early psychological and pharmacological intervention after traumatic events. Journal of Psychosocial Nursing 2003;41:42–51.

[15] Bisson J, Deahl M. Psychological debriefing and prevention of post-traumatic stress. More research is needed. Br J Psychiatry 1994;165:717–20.

[16] Solomon SD, Davidson JRT. Trauma: prevalence, impairment, service, use, and cost. J Clin Psychiatry 1997;58:5–11.

[17] Summerfield D. The invention of post-traumatic stress disorder and the social usefulness of a psychiatric category. BMJ 2001;322:95–8.

[18] DeWolfe DJ. Training manual for mental health and human service workers in major disasters. Washington (DC), US Department of Human Services, ADM publication #90–538.

[19] Plum KC. Understanding the psychosocial impact of disasters. In: Veenema TG, editor. Disaster and Emergency preparedness for chemical, biological, radiological terrorism and other hazards. New York: Springer Publishing; 2003. p. 63–81.

[20] Townsend MJ. Psychiatric mental health nursing: concepts of care. 2nd edition. Philadelphia: FA Davis; 1996.

[21] Davidson JR, Hughes DB, Blazer DG. Post-traumatic stress disorder in the community: an epidemiological study. Psychol Med 1991;21:713–21.

[22] Kessler R, Sonnega A, Bromet E, et al. Posttraumatic stress disorder in the national comorbidity survey. Arch Gen Psychiatry 1995;52:1048–60.

[23] Mitchell JT, Everly GS. Critical incident stress debriefing (CISD): an operations manual for the prevention of traumatic stress among emergency services and disaster workers. 2nd edition. Ellicott City (MD): Chevron Publishing; 1996.

[24] Plum KC, Veenema TG. Management of psychosocial effects. In: Veenema TG, editor. Disaster and emergency preparedness for chemical, biological, and radiological terrorism and other hazards. New York NY: Springer Publishing; 2003. p. 203–19.

[25] National Institute of Mental Health. Mental health and mass violence: evidence-based early psychological intervention for victims/survivors of mass violence. A Workshop to Reach Consensus on Best Practices, 2002. Washington (DC), US Government Printing Office, NIH publication #02–5138.NIH.

[26] van Etten ML, Taylor S. Comparative efficacy of treatment for post-traumatic disorder: a meta-analysis. J Trauma Stress 1998;11:413–36.

[27] Adshead G. Psychological therapies for post-traumatic stress disorder. Br J Psychiatry 2000;177:144–8.

[28] Shapiro F. Eye movement desensitization: a new treatment for post-traumatic stress disorder. J Behav Ther Exp Psychiatry 1989;20:211–7.

[29] Mitchell JT. When disaster strikes...the critical incident stress debriefing process. Journal of Emergency Medical Services (JEMS) 1983;8(1):36–9.

[30] Everly GS, Boyle SH. Critical incident debriefing (CISD): a meta-analysis. Int J Emerg Mental Health 1999;3:165–8.

[31] Rose S, Wessley S, Bisson J. Brief psychological interventions (debriefing) for trauma-related symptoms and prevention of posttraumatic stress disorder. Cochrane Database Syst Rev 2001;1–30.

[32] van Emmerik AA, Kamphuis JH, Hulsbosch AM, et al. Single session debriefing after psychological trauma: a meta-analysis. Lancet 2002;360:766–71.

[33] Flannery RB, Everly GS. Crisis intervention: a review. Int J Emerg Mental Health 2000;2:119–25.

[34] Bisson J. Post-traumatic stress disorder. In: Barton S, editor. Clinical evidence: the international source of the best available evidence for effective health care. 5th edition. London: BMJ Publishing; 2001. p. 688–94.

[35] Richards D. A field study of critical incident stress debriefing versus critical incident stress management. Journal of Mental Health 2001;10:351–62.

[36] Litz BT, Gray MJ, Bryant RA. Early intervention for trauma: current status and future directions. Clin Psychol 2002;9:112–34.

[37] Bisson JI, McFarlane AC, Rose A. Psychological debriefing. In: Foa EB, Keane TM, editors. Effective treatment for PTSD. New York: Guilford Press; 2000. p. 39–59.

[38] Katz LK, Fleisher W, Kjernisted K, et al. A review pf the psychobiology and pharmacology of post-traumatic stress disorder. Can J Psychiatry 1996;41:233–8.

[39] Stein DJ, Seedat S, van der Linden GH, et al. Selective serotonin reuptake inhibitors in the treatment of post-traumatic disorder: a meta-analysis of randomized controlled trials. Int Clin Psychopharmacol 2000;15(Suppl 2):s31–9.

[40] Rivas-Vazquez RA, Saffer-Biller D, Ruiz I, et al. Current issues in anxiety and depression: comorbid, mixed, and subthreshold disorders. Prof Psychol Res Pr 2004;35(1):74–83.

[41] Rivas-Vazquez RA. Benzodiazepines in contemporary clinical practice. Prof Psychol Res Pr 2003;34(3):324–8.

[42] Asnis GM, Kohn SR, Henderson M, et al. SSRIs versus non-SSRIs in post-traumatic stress disorder: An update with recommendations. Drugs 2004;64(4):383–404.

Nurs Clin N Am 40 (2005) 551–564

NURSING CLINICS
OF NORTH AMERICA

Research Issues in Preparedness for Mass Casualty Events, Disaster, War, and Terrorism

Patricia Hinton Walker, PhD, RN, FAAN*,
Sandra C. Garmon Bibb, DNSc, RN,
Karen L. Elberson, PhD, RN

Graduate School of Nursing, Uniformed Services University of the Health Sciences,
4301 Jones Bridge Road, Bethesda, MD 20814, USA

Conducting research that focuses on preparedness for mass casualty events, disaster, war, and terrorism presents significant ethical, legal, and scientific challenges. Little research has been reported in this area, largely because of difficulties in obtaining subjects, collecting data, the timing of the research endeavor in relation to the occurrence of an event, and the sensitivity required to deal with disaster victims. Research by military nurses has produced data on wartime situations that has applicability to emergency preparedness. To improve care and prevent repeated mistakes, the importance of conducting research in the midst of and subsequent to disasters and mass casualty events cannot be overstated.

Like research on many other health-related topics, the purpose of research conducted relative to mass casualty events is ultimately to ensure and measure quality of health care provided and delivered in these unusual types of situations. For this very necessary research to take place, nurses and members of other disciplines must plan proactively to seize opportunities for conducting research at all stages of these events: preparedness, response, and recovery. Proactive planning requires the thinking through of strategies for timely initiation and management of research studies should disasters such as those that took place on September 11, 2001, re-occur.

This article provides a perspective on the types of research questions that might be explored and strategies used in relation to disaster, terrorism, and mass casualty events. Research is addressed in the context of three areas of focus: issues related to the health care provider; issues affecting the patient, individual, family, and community; and issues related to the health care system. Within this context, researchers (nurse scientists and those from other

*Corresponding author. E-mail address: phintonwalker@usuhs.mil (P. Hinton Walker).

0029-6465/05/$ – see front matter
doi:10.1016/j.cnur.2005.04.008

disciplines) interested in prospective and retrospective research projects should be able to design studies that ultimately improve care during mass casualty events. In such research endeavors, emphasis must be placed on legal and ethical issues in regards to sensitivity extended not only to disaster victims, their significant others, and community members, but also to health care providers and other public servants, including fire fighters and law enforcement. Whereas those injured or sickened are recognized as victims of disaster, all too often members of the disaster response team (health care providers and others) are overlooked. Awareness of this oversight is imperative when considering the complexities of the situation and the overarching impact of casualties on all involved. Thus, researchers should observe for the likelihood of post-traumatic stress responses in all victims and potential victims.

Because of the nature of research problems in disaster, an evaluation-related research approach seems the most likely because of significant challenges in gaining access to subjects, developing a realistic research design, and collecting data. Ideally, prospective studies with stringent research designs are the preferred approach; however, retrospective research protocols are the method used historically. Thus, the challenges of conducting research related to bioterrorism and mass casualty events are addressed. In addition, a brief overview of research that has been conducted or is currently funded related to this effort is described.

CHALLENGES IN CONDUCTING RESEARCH RELATED TO MASS CASUALTY EVENTS, DISASTER, AND TERRORISM

The conduct of research addressing problems related to mass casualty events, disaster and terrorism, is an important area for research by nurse scientists. Types of research needed include: basic science (bench) research, development of reliable instrumentation, demonstration research projects on preparedness, intervention research (for both providers and clients), and health services research designed to evaluate and enhance systems-level response and recovery stages of mass casualty events. Nurse scientists are advised that they will face significant legal, ethical and scientific challenges previously identified by researchers in disaster medicine. Given the chaotic nature of bioterrorism and mass casualty events, these challenges to the conduct of good science are to be expected and must be considered carefully. Examples of these challenges include: development of a sound, scientific study that protects study subjects and researchers while clearly achieving important and measurable research objectives; identification and recruitment of subjects from an extremely vulnerable population base; addressing timely data collection in the context of ethical and legal consideration; attempting to conduct research in sometimes threatening and difficult environments; and attention to maintenance of objectivity in highly emotionally charged research settings [1]. Importantly, research conducted by nurse scientists should have the breadth needed to address issues related not only to patient/community needs and safety and preparedness of providers, but also to issues surrounding effective planning, training, and improvement of the quality of care within the health system.

To protect the public and address complex health system issues, a research agenda should include strategies for improving communication and collaboration between and among provider organizations and communities. Research issues of this nature need further exploration. Exploration could result in policy change, not only for the public, but also for provider groups. Thus, nurse scientists have significant opportunity for planning and conducting research that addresses provider issues and safety.

Research conducted by interdisciplinary groups has great potential for informing nurse scientists in terms of topics, research design and methods. Research done in the past by nurses and others in disaster management underscores the value of retrospective research. To have significant impact on mitigation and preparedness, and response and recovery, prospective research must be initiated. To play a part in developing the necessary health services research at the systems level, nurses have an imperative to participate in the evaluation science of planning, exercises, and response to virtual and actual disaster situations. A collaborative approach between nurse scientists and other interdisciplinary colleagues is needed to conduct the complex research necessary to improve care in bioterrorism and mass casualty events. Nurse researchers have qualitative, quantitative and health services research methodological expertise required to address the complexities of research questions that need to be explored.

Nurses should be leaders in identifying how nursing research can inform practice, education, health systems delivery, and health policy in this emerging area of research. Since the events of September 11, 2001, recognition of the need for preparedness and improving the competency of emergency responders, including nurses, has grown exponentially. Communities will continue to depend upon health care providers, including nurses, for guidance, education, and advocacy when a mass casualty event occurs.

WHY IS THIS RESEARCH AGENDA IMPORTANT?

Why is this topic such an important research agenda item for the nursing profession and for nurse scientists? Nurses with all levels of preparation are key to improving management of disasters at home and abroad. Nurses are recognized as vital health care resources in their neighborhoods and communities. Nurses work effectively on interdisciplinary teams and improvise readily when situations call for flexible thinking and innovation. Historically, the nursing profession has advocated for preventive approaches, not only to disease and health care, but in disaster planning and training. Nurses will continue to play critical roles in disaster mitigation and preparedness. Further, the integration of care related to psychological, social support and family-oriented issues, in addition to physiological needs of patients, is an important part of the nursing model of care. Although diminishing in numbers because of the nursing shortage, many practicing and retired nurses would be available should health care needs arise in their own communities. The recognition of nurses as key health care resources re-emphasizes the value of conducting research related not only to the role of nurses as providers and the impact of nursing on patients, but also on health care delivery systems.

CATEGORIZATION OF RESEARCH AND FUNDING
Research related to mass casualty events, disaster, war, and terrorism can be categorized into three areas: (1) studies related to the training, preparedness, and safety of providers along with the impact of mass casualty events on provider mental health; (2) studies related to patients (individuals, families, and communities); and (3) studies related to communication and collaboration in the context of response and recovery by health care delivery systems. Little research by civilian groups was found; however, a growing body of knowledge generated by military researchers has emerged. Before September 11, 2001, these studies did not seem relevant to terrorism and mass casualty response, but with the growth of homeland security initiatives, the applicability to the understanding of the roles and preparation of nurses as providers in mass casualty events can be seen. The body of research conducted in wartime and in war-effected environments is now relevant.

RESEARCH RELATED TO PROVIDERS
Unstructured interviews and field study approaches have focused mostly on providers with little research addressing the needs of the patient (individuals, family victims, or communities). In the nursing literature, the focus of many studies has been on personal accounts of nurses. Some of the first research related to nursing's role in disasters was in identification of the stressors of health care workers during and after the event. Bell [2] conducted and disseminated research related to stressors and changes in health outcomes of women in the Persian Gulf War. Given the experiences of rescuers and health care providers reported in the news media from the Oklahoma City bombing and the attacks of September 11, 2001, a need for more research related to the short- and long-term impact of terrorism on health care workers exists.

RELEVANCE OF MILITARY NURSING RESEARCH
Although studies documenting the history of the Army and Air Force Nurse Corps may not seem relevant to current nursing research issues, they offer insight into the wartime experiences of nurses as providers. These historical studies reflect relevant issues such as preparation requirements, emotional reactions, and nursing challenges from World War I, World War II, the Korean War, and the Vietnam War. Several studies highlight challenges related to preparation requirements including: a comprehensive history of the Army Nurse Corps from its origins through the period of the Vietnam War by Sarnecky [3], accounts of the hardships and experiences of nurses in Vietnam following their adjustments as female veterans by Scannell-Desch [4], interviews of nurses who served in Vietnam and those nurses imprisoned on

Bataan during World War II by Norman [5], and current historical documentation of the Air Force Nurse Corps by Smolenski [6]. Similar issues have emerged in the documentation of activation, preparation, and readiness in OPERATION DESERT SHIELD/DESERT STORM in work by Agazio and Gurney [7], Gurney [8], and Nelson [9].

These studies are important, but as important is the preparation of providers and citizens for possible terror attack. Skill sustainment training and readiness competency research are crucial to self-preservation of civilians and military providers and is necessary for delivering quality care.

Components associated with readiness competency were defined by Reineck, who subsequently developed and tested an instrument to assess individual readiness [10–13]. Research that focused upon specific skill retention includes: trauma skills (Driscoll [14], Pierce [15], Topley [16]), readiness-related factors (Sisk [17]), retention of BCLS/ACLS skills (Smith [18]), and triage knowledge (Janousek [19]). Dorn [20], Johnson [21], and Page [22] focused their research on optimal training methods to affect retention of critical readiness skills. Also, in a funded research project, Sykes sought to increase readiness of Air Force active duty and reserve nurses using a Web-based computer-assisted training program and simulation laboratory [23].

Progress made in this area is evidenced by the fact that the current literature informs future directions for a nursing research agenda for individual providers, for the educational systems that teach and train current and future providers, and for patients/families and communities. Significant work has been accomplished by Gebbie [24] and the International Nursing Coalition for Mass Casualty Education (INCMCE) [25] in developing core competencies for nurses. As health care delivery systems and community leaders develop disaster plans, the importance of building on prior relevant research studies, specifically those related to readiness competencies and the sustainment of readiness, cannot be overemphasized. Belfort [26], with the New York State Department of Health, received funding to develop a program to provide multi-disciplinary training combining basic and applied research in an effort to produce doctoral graduates with competencies in dealing with biodefense and emerging infectious disease and postdoctoral fellows as independent scientists whose research programs integrate biodefense and emerging infections. Additionally, Dembry [27], of the Connecticut State Department of Public Health, has a funded project that is focused on identifying specific training programs for front-line clinicians and on evaluating program effectiveness. Further, Green [28], of Johns Hopkins University, received funding to develop and apply techniques that are supported by evidence-based expert consensus to create and operationalize standard best practice course content for training clinicians in bioterrorism and disaster response.

Another major area of research conducted by military nurses is related to provider safety in the context of changes in the bio–chemical environment. Research considering the implications of providing care while garbed in protective clothing during possible bio–chemical mass casualty situations in the

United States are particularly relevant to the threats of bio–chemical attacks and the postanthrax scare. Studies concerning Mission Oriented Protective Posture (MOPP) gear refer to a stratification of different levels of protection that are available for providers currently [29]. The level is dictated by the anticipated magnitude and type of threat from chemical or biological agents. These five levels range from 0 to 4, with 0 being the least protective. MOPP equipment consists of overgarment and helmet cover, vinyl overboot, mask and hood, and gloves. At MOPP 0, military personnel carry protective masks and hoods and have the rest of the gear available for use within a 2-hour time frame. At MOPP 1, the overgarment and helmet cover are worn; the masks and hood and gloves are carried, and the vinyl overboots are available. At MOPP 2, the overgarment, helmet cover, and vinyl overboots are worn, and the masks and hood and gloves are carried. At MOPP 3, gloves are carried and the remainder of the gear is worn. At MOPP 4, all gear is worn. MOPP 4 provides the highest degree of chemical protection and at the same time creates a major challenge because of the limits protective garments place on the individual's ability to perform. This negative impact is the result of the physical burden of bulky and heavy fully protective gear that increases the risk of heat stress and potential for dehydration. Additionally, cumbersome boots impede the ability to walk and increase the risk of falls. Also, greater than usual fatigue from the weight of the full gear is likely to occur.

Agazio [30] conducted research to determine whether increased difficulty in providing nursing care occurs when nurses wear MOPP 4. This researcher evaluated the use of a virtual reality simulator for sustainment training in IV insertion skills while in bio–chemical protective gloves and clothing. Using a simulator, Agazio found that IV insertion performance is impaired significantly by the restriction of the heavy gloves and decreased visual field. A static IV arm associated with a virtual reality simulator provided a good model for practice of IV insertion under research conditions. Different patient scenarios were provided to make the exercise more interesting and less personally burdensome. This research is an example of opportunities that exist to use simulations, standardized patients, and virtual environments to test and evaluate the competencies and performance of providers and in certain cases even patients in future disaster and bioterrorism situations.

Another research study related to the use of MOPP gear during military training was conducted by Johnson and Schmelz [31]. They investigated the most effective product (power drink, fruit-flavored glucose drink, or water) for maintaining fluid and electrolyte balance and blood sugar levels in individuals wearing MOPP gear. Whereas fluid and electrolytes were maintained with water during MOPP training, these researchers found that the use of the power drink decreased perceptions of fatigue, perhaps because of the glucose content. More research in this area related to fluid and electrolyte balance and dehydration is needed.

Another area of research related to fluid management was conducted by military nurse scientists focusing on female health care providers and female military personnel. Ryan-Wenger [32] and Czerwinski [33] focused on women's needs, specifically gynecological and urological health of deployed women. They were the first to describe the need for modification in hygienic practices. They documented health care needs in the field, and then developed and tested field sanitation kits. More recently, Criner was funded to investigate the influences of field barriers to incontinence and examine psychosocial impact symptom distress of stress urinary incontinence on military women in the field [34]. This research has implications for women and nurses involved in disaster situations, where response and recovery are not resolved in a short period of time.

RESEARCH RELATED TO PATIENT, FAMILY, AND COMMUNITY

Heightened awareness of the possibility of terrorism attack within the United States makes exploration and building on the current state of the science extremely important. Although few studies conducted by civilian nurses can be found in the literature, military nurses have been active in research in this area. Research has focused on the role, needs, and safety of nurses as providers. Compared with research related to provider's needs, a minimal amount of research related to patient, family, and community issues and needs conducted by nurse scientists was found.

Research conducted on the patient, family, and community is comprised primarily of qualitative studies describing lived experiences. Historical studies conducted by military nurse researchers offer a grounding in the wartime experience through the use of first-person narrative analysis or review of source documents [35–37]. Similar methodologies were used here as were used in the previously mentioned studies conducted by civilian nurses in postdisaster periods. The ethical and legal challenges of getting timely access to patients and families, however, make this an important area for future planning and consideration. Not surprisingly, little research and literature exist in this area.

Nursing research projects conducted by Ryan-Wenger [38] were undertaken to study the impact of the threat of war upon military children. Messecar [39] investigated family stress associated with wartime separation, and Birgenheier [40,41] studied another family issue, the impact of military parent's separation on children. With long deployments of active duty, reserve, and National Guard personnel, such research is particularly relevant. Additionally, in a study funded by the TriService Nursing Research Program (TSNRP), Russek [42] explored the resiliency in Army reserve families before deployment. One of the more promising areas of research has been conducted by Schoneboom [43]. One of few nurse scientists considering specific biological threats to the health of the public, Schoneboom characterized early immune responses of glial cells to Venezuelan equine encephalitis (VEE) virus infection. Although VEE is endemic to parts of South America, this viral pathogen has potential to be weaponized. Schoneboom found that VEE infection in glial cells in mice caused significant pathology, especially related to the virulence of the VEE strain. This research has implications for understanding the means to develop and provide host protection and treatment in the event of an attack using a virus or other similar pathogen.

The National Institute of Allergy and Infectious Diseases (NIAID) [44] outlined plans to address bioterrorism and emerging and re-emerging diseases. According to NIAID, basic research on microbe biology, host response, and research that focuses on developing diagnostics, therapeutics, and vaccine against these agents is imperative. Given these needs, Liu [45] was funded to conduct a series of annual meetings for sharing information directed toward solving bioterrorism issues. Among the aims that Liu outlined was the attraction of young scientists who would develop their program of research around biodefense. A final aim of these proposed symposia is to ultimately provide the setting for providing effective ideas for managing the bioterrorism threat.

Since September 11, 2001, Americans feel an increased vulnerability to terrorism that includes acts of war such as use of biological and chemical agents. Previous research conducted by military nurses lends an initial understanding of nursing practice in austere environments, primarily during wartime. Less research, however, can be found related to biochemical defense for the patient and provider under similar conditions. More research is needed so that nurses and other health care providers can enhance prevention, host protection, and provide clinical interventions that aim to save lives of patients, families, and communities in future bioterrorism situations.

RESEARCH ON HEALTH SYSTEMS ISSUES

Research related to health systems response also is limited. Nurses, as one of the largest groups of health care providers, need to be used effectively and efficiently in disaster response. Early researchers Demi and Miles [46] reported a lack of integration of nurses in the planning and subsequently in the response as key areas for ongoing research. Rivera, in describing the response to the Mexico earthquake [47], noted confusion because of lack of guidelines for use of nurses, physicians, and medications. Further, Rivera identified the need for educational institutions to prepare nurses for disasters in coordination with local agencies such as the American Red Cross. Nurse scientists should conduct research that focuses on ways nurses can be used better. Research priorities include the determination of appropriate educational preparation for readiness and research on communication and coordination activities among local and national response agencies [48].

A separate category of military nursing research literature addresses nursing care delivery with health systems implications. Descriptive studies have been conducted on nursing practice in humanitarian missions or operations other than war [49], the experience of chief nurses in nonwar military operations [50], shipboard practice environment [51,52], and advanced practice nurses and flight nursing [53]. Bridges [54] and Schmelz [55] developed an ongoing program of aeromedical nursing research. These studies include specific nursing care practices and topics such as: prevention of hypoxemia from suctioning at high altitudes, considerations related to litter placement during air transport, and implications for skin pressure and cardiopulmonary resuscitation using the NATO litter for evacuation [56]. In a study funded by the TriService Nursing Research Program (TSNRP), Dremsa [57] initiated research to describe knowledge gained by critical care air transport team nurses while providing patient care in a combat environment.

These studies provide important contributions for health systems research and not only address implications for the research agenda of nurses, but also for other providers. Also, such research is relevant in identifying and addressing the challenges of emergency response teams and their need to plan for evacuation of patients and families in future bioterrorism or disaster situations.

From a health systems perspective, the appropriate use of nurses is important in effective disaster response. According to Hinton Walker and colleagues [48], because of the changing nature of the threats related to bioterrorism, approaches to mass immunization and mass medication distribution need to be explored. Demonstration research projects should be designed and conducted that include all health professions, particularly nurses in training exercises between and among health care systems, communities, and government agencies. Models need to be tested and validated in urban and rural settings where advance practice nurses (APNs) are likely to be primary care providers to vulnerable populations. Unfortunately, one of the challenges in many of the disaster plans and training exercises is that vulnerable populations (pediatric, elderly, and those with English as a second language) may be more at risk because of inadequate plans for communication, evacuation, and care issues. Equally unfortunate is the concern that nurses who care for many of these populations may not be sufficiently effective in influencing health systems planning. Nurse researchers, whose studies historically have focused on care of vulnerable populations and issues related to lack of access to services, need to be involved not only in setting the research agenda for the future, but also in the conduct of the research in this important area.

Other health systems issues include the impact of mass casualty events on the financial health of health care delivery systems. For example, during the events of September 11, 2001, some hospitals evacuated patients who were not critically ill and cancelled elective surgery to prepare to receive casualties, but fewer casualties than expected arrived. Loss of revenue and possible costs of treating the underinsured and uninsured populations are issues to be considered in similar circumstances. Health services research projects and the issue of providing access to care for vulnerable populations has been a long-standing interest of nurse researchers. For example, how does one balance the need for provision of free care and services in a bioterrorism event outside the boundaries of collecting dollars through the traditional insurance industry? How does one justify the costs to the private sector or the federal government for free care in the presence of a moral/ethical responsibility of ensuring the health of the public? These ethical, legal, and financial issues can be addressed by creating and testing predictive models in advance of future bioterrorism and disaster situations [48].

Examples of currently funded research focusing on systems are applications of modeling and simulation informatics to enhance homeland security and readiness [58]; a project that promotes bioterrorism and public health emergency preparedness [59]; assessment of improvements in linkages between health care organizations, the public health infrastructure, and emergency response entities relative to the revised Joint Commission on the Accreditation of Health care Organizations (JCAHO) emergency management standards, occurrence of national events, and federal funding [60]; development of mathematical models related to the transmission and within-host dynamics of bioterrorism agents or naturally occurring infectious diseases that can be validated and implemented [61]; and assessment of US hospital capacity for bioterrorism and public health emergency response using advanced computer modeling techniques [62]. These studies relate to systems, resource allocation and distribution, and safety of the workforce and victims of bioterrorism or natural disasters.

THE TRISERVICE NURSING RESEARCH PROGRAM

Active duty, retired military nurses, and reservists have contributed to research related to disaster, bioterrorism, and wartime casualty care because of the funding of the TSNRP. The TSNRP provides resources for research that fosters excellence in military nursing care. One major goal of the program is to expand the breadth, depth, and promulgation of research related to deployment health. Six deployment-related studies received funding from TSNRP in 2004. Hopkins was funded to study motherhood, stress, and role strain in junior enlisted women [63]. Pierce was funded to examine the multiple and interactive effects of war-related stressors that impact the physical and mental health and retention of women in the armed forces [64]. Ross [65] was funded to examine the use of after action reports for readiness competency training, and Rivers [66] was funded to study the perceived readiness of professional filler personnel in relation to competency and readiness for deployment. Finally, McNulty [67] was funded to study deployed families and their health needs, and Williams was funded to conduct a follow-up intervention study that identifies/describes coping strategies related to mental health issues in Navy personnel [68].

FUTURE DIRECTIONS

Future nursing research agenda not only must address provider issues that include preparation, readiness, and protection, but also must focus on client and health care system outcomes. Because nurses traditionally have focused on patient or client advocacy and education for health promotion and prevention, nurse scientists should be the first to expand research conducted related to patients, families, and communities and research related to health systems.

Two clear directions for the future include research focused on the client's needs at the individual and community level and on significant approaches to health policy issues. Knowledge of APNs who provide primary care in disaster needs to be assessed. Building on work accomplished primarily by military nurses, research needs to be conducted that explores how technology (simulation, virtual environments, standardized patients, and the Internet) can be used to educate nurses, patients, families, communities, and health systems to prepare for disasters and bioterrorism.

With the continued threat of terrorism, another area ripe for research is the need to examine and improve the health care consumer's awareness, preparation, and education. Nurses are in a unique position to provide care to patients across the health care continuum. Opportunities abound for practice-based research initiatives in public health departments; primary care clinics; and in acute care, long-term care, and school-based care settings.

Nurse scientists must consider health policy implications and the ethics of individual decision-making for individuals and communities versus governmental decision-making. Differing cultural perspectives and values from communities need to be explored to appropriately shape health policy decisions for an increasingly diverse population. In the context of national security and population health, a need exists for qualitative and quantitative research addressing the balance of the patient's voice and input into public policy decisions versus the need to ensure the health of the public in terrorism and disaster situations.

Progress has been made in exploring preparedness for disaster, terrorism, war, and disaster; however, only the surface of these areas has been scratched. Work done in the military sector should be replicated in the civilian sector and should be moved to the next level of research. The issue is not only that the nursing profession and nurse scientists step up to the challenge, but also that private and public sector funding sources identify funding to address the needs for research described in this article.

References
[1] Quick G, Hogan DE. Research in disaster medicine. In: Hogan D, Burstein JL, editors. Disaster medicine. Philadelphia: Lippincott, Williams & Wilkins; 2002. p. 395–403.
[2] Bell E. Wartime stressors and health outcomes: women in the Persian Gulf War. J Psychosoc Nurs Ment Health Serv 1998;36:19–25.
[3] Sarnecky M. A history of the Army Nurse Corps [abstract]. Available at: http://www.usuhs.mil/tsnrp/funded/fy1993/sarnecky.html. Accessed September 14, 2004.
[4] Scannell-Desch E. The lived experience of women military nurses in Vietnam during the Vietnam War. Image J Nurs Sch 1996;28:119–24.
[5] Norman E. We band of angels: the untold story of American women trapped on Bataan by the Japanese. Nurs News 1999;49(4):6–7.
[6] Smolenski M. A history of the US Air Force Nursing Service [abstract]. Available at: http://www.usuhs.mil/tsnrp/funded/fy1999/smolenski.html. Accessed September 9, 2004.
[7] Agazio J, Gurney C. Through the eyes of the medic: Operation Desert Storm. US Army Medical Department Journal 2001; October-December: 16–23.
[8] Gurney C. Adaptation of medical personnel to combat. US Army Medical Department Journal 2001; October-December: 8–16.

[9] Nelson B. Activation experiences during the Persian Gulf War [abstract]. Available at: http://www.usuhs.mil/tsnrp/funded/fy1994/nelson.html. Accessed September 14, 2004.

[10] Reineck C. Readiness instrument psychometric evaluation [abstract]. Available at: http://www.usuhs.mil/tsnrp/funded/fy1998/reineck.html. Accessed September 14, 2004.

[11] Reineck C. Individual medical readiness: concept clarification [abstract]. Available at: http://www.usuhs.mil/tsnrp/funded/fy1996/reineck.html. Accessed September 14, 2004.

[12] Reineck C. Individual readiness in nursing: the Federal Nursing Service Award. Mil Med 1999;164(4):251–5.

[13] Reineck C, Finstuen K, Connelly LM, et al. Army nurse readiness instrument: psychometric evaluation and field administration. Mil Med 2001;166(11):931–9.

[14] Driscoll D. Nursing retention of trauma resuscitative skills [abstract]. Available at: http://www.usuhs.mil/tsnrp/funded/fy2001/driscoll.html. Accessed September 14, 2004.

[15] Pierce P. Identification of trauma skills for nursing personnel [abstract]. Available at: http://www.usuhs.mil/tsnrp/funded/fy1999/pierce.html. Accessed September 14, 2004.

[16] Topley D. Critical care nursing expertise during air transport [abstract]. Available at: http://www.usuhs.mil/tsnrp/funded/fy1997/topley.html. Accessed September 14, 2004.

[17] Sisk R. Related to medical readiness in military reservists [abstract]. Available at: http://www.usuhs.mil/tsnrp/funded/fy1997/sisk.html. Accessed September 14, 2004.

[18] Smith K. Evaluation of staff's retention of BCLS and ACLS skills [abstract]. Available at: http://www.usuhs.mil/tsnrp/funded/fy1999/smith.html. Accessed September 9, 2004.

[19] Janousek JT, Jackson DE, De Lorenzo RA, et al. Mass casualty triage knowledge of military medical personnel. Mil Med 1999;164(5):332–5.

[20] Dorn D. Dietary and exercise intervention to improve readiness [abstract]. Available at: http://www.usuhs.mil/tsnrp/funded/fy1999/dorn.html. Accessed September 14, 2004.

[21] Johnson A. Effects of 3 fluids on hydration during MOPP training [abstract]. Available at: http://www.usuhs.mil/tsnrp/funded/fy1997/johnsonb.html. Accessed September 14, 2004.

[22] Page N. Development of an advanced life support patient transfer training program. Mil Med 2000;165(11):821–3.

[23] Sykes C. Wartime competencies for the USAF nurse: training for sustainment [abstract]. Available at: http://www.usuhs.mil/tsnrp/funded/fy1999/sykes.html. Accessed September 14, 2004.

[24] Gebbie K. Preparing currently employed public health professionals for changes in the health systems. New York: Columbia University School of Nursing, Center for Health Policy; 1998. Available at: http://www.nursing.hs.columbia.edu/institute-centers/chphsr/publications.html. Accessed September 14, 2004.

[25] International Nursing Coalition for Mass Casualty Education (INCMCE). Educational competencies for registered nurses responding to mass casualty incidents. Nashville (TN): INCMCE Competency Committee; 2003. Available at: http://www.aacn.nche.edu/Education/INCMCECompetencies.pdf. Accessed September 14, 2004.

[26] Belfort M. Training in biodefense and emerging infectious disease [abstract]. Available at: http://crisp.cit.nih.gov/crisp/crisp_query.generate_screen. Accessed September 14, 2004.

[27] Dembry L. Training for improved provider response to bioterrorism [abstract]. Available at: http://crisp.cit.nih.gov/crisp/crisp_query.generate_screen. Accessed September 14, 2004.

[28] Green G. Evaluation of bioterrorism training for clinicians [abstract]. Available at: http://crisp.cit.nih.gov/crisp/crisp_query.generate_screen. Accessed September 14, 2004.

[29] Rostker B. Mission oriented protective posture (MOPP) and chemical protection: information paper. Available at: http://www.gulflink.osd.mil/mopp/mopp. Accessed September 14, 2004.

[30] Agazio J. Evaluation of a virtual reality simulator in sustainment training [abstract]. Available at: http://www.usuhs.mil/tsnrp/funded/fy1999/agazio.html. Accessed September 14, 2004.

[31] Johnson A. Effects of 3 fluids on hydration during MOPP training [abstract]. Available at: http://www.usuhs.mil/tsnrp/funded/fy1997/johnsonb.html. Accessed September 14, 2004.

[32] Ryan-Wenger N. GYN self-care and military women in austere environments [abstract]. Available at: http://www.usuhs.mil/tsnrp/funded/fy1996/wenger.html. Accessed September 14, 2004.

[33] Czerwinski BS, Wardell DW, Yoder LH, et al. Variations in feminine hygiene practices of military women deployed and noncombat environments. Mil Med 2001;166(2):152–8.

[34] Criner J. Coping stages by military women with stress urinary incontinence [abstract]. Available at: http://www.usuhs.mil/tsnrp/funded/fy2003/criner.html. Accessed September 14, 2004.

[35] Dittmar SS, Stanton MP, Jezewski MA, et al. Images and sensations of war: a common theme in the history of military nursing. Health Care Women Int 1996;17(1):69–80.

[36] Stanton MP, Dittmar SS, Jezewski MA, et al. Shared experiences and meanings of military nurse veterans. Image J Nurs Sch 1996;28(4):343–7.

[37] Stanton-Bandiero MP, Jezewski MA, Dickerson SS. The war experience for nurse veterans: a secondary data analysis. Journal of Military Nursing and Research 1996;2(1):12–7.

[38] Ryan-Wenger N. Impact of the threat of war on military children [abstract]. Available at: http://www.usuhs.mil/tsnrp/funded/fy1994/wenger.html. Accessed September 14, 2004.

[39] Messecar D. Family stress associated with wartime separation [abstract]. Available at: http://www.usuhs.mil/tsnrp/funded/fy1993/messecar.html. Accessed September 14, 2004.

[40] Birgenheier P. Effects of military parents' separation on children [abstract]. Available at: http://www.usuhs.mil/tsnrp/funded/fy1993/birgen.html. Accessed September 14, 2004.

[41] Birgenheier P. Parents and children: war and separation. Journal of Military Nursing Research 1995;1(3):30–3, 45.

[42] Russek JA. Resiliency in Army Reserve families before deployment [abstract]. Available at: http://www.usuhs.mil/tsnrp/funded/fy2003/russek.html. Accessed September 14, 2004.

[43] Schoneboom B. Neuro–immune responses of astrocytes following alphavirus infection [abstract]. Available at: http://www.usuhs.mil/tsnrp/funded/fy1998/schboom.html. Accessed September 14, 2004.

[44] National Institute of Allergy and Infectious Diseases (NIAID). Available at: http://www2.niaid.nih.gov/Biodefense/Research/strat_plan.htm; http://www2.niaid.nih.gov/Biodefense/Research/funding.htm#B. Accessed September 14, 2004.

[45] Liu MA. Biodefense initiative: Connecting biodefense community [abstract]. Available at: http://crisp.cit.nih.gov/crisp/crisp_query.generate_screen. Accessed September 14, 2004.

[46] Demi AS, Miles MS. An examination of nursing leadership following a disaster. Top Clin Nurs 1984;6(1):63–78.

[47] Anonymous. Mexico earthquake. Int Nurs Rev 1986;33(4):125–6.

[48] Hinton Walker P, Ricciardi R, Agazio J. Directions for nursing research and development. In: Veenema T, editor. Disaster nursing and emergency preparedness for chemical, biological and radiological terrorism and other hazards. New York: Springer Publishing Company; 2003. p. 473–84.

[49] Shafer M. Nurses during deployment to Croatia: a grounded theory [abstract]. Available at: http://www.usuhs.mil/tsnrp/funded/fy1996/shafer.html. Accessed September 14, 2004.

[50] Turner D. Experience of chief nurses in non-war military operations [abstract]. Available at: http://www.usuhs.mil/tsnrp/funded/fy1997/turnerd.html. Accessed September 14, 2004.

[51] Connor-Ballard P. Angels of the Mercy Fleet: Nursing the ill & wounded aboard US Navy hospital ships in the Pacific during World War II [abstract]. Available at: http://www.usuhs.mil/tsnrp/funded/fy1998/connor.html. Accessed September 14, 2004.

[52] Cox C. The lived experience of nurses stationed aboard aircraft carriers [abstract]. Available at: http://www.usuhs.mil/tsnrp/funded/fy2000/cox.html. Accessed September 14, 2004.

[53] Chamings P. Flight nursing and the US Air Force Nurse Corps [abstract]. Available at: http://www.usuhs.mil/tsnrp/funded/fy1994/chamings.html. Accessed September 14, 2004.

[54] Bridges E. Invasive pressure monitoring in aeromedical evacuation [abstract]. Available at: http://www.usuhs.mil/tsnrp/funded/fy2002/bridges.html. Accessed September 14, 2004.

[55] Schmelz J. Preventing suctioning-induced hypoxemia at altitude [abstract]. Available at: http://www.usuhs.mil/tsnrp/funded/fy1998/schmelz.html. Accessed September 14, 2004.

[56] Bridges E. Efficacy of cardiopulmonary resuscitation in the field: effect of the NATO litter with and without a backboard [abstract]. Available at: http://www.usuhs.mil/tsnrp/funded/fy2001/bridges.html. Accessed September 14, 2004.

[57] Dremsa T. CCATT nurses' deployed experience [abstract]. Available at: http://www.usuhs.mil/tsnrp/funded/. Accessed September 14, 2004.

[58] Miller G. Improving healthcare responses to bioterrorist events [abstract]. Available at: http://crisp.cit.nih.gov/crisp/crisp_query.generate_screen. Accessed September 14, 2004.

[59] Dobalian A. Bioterrorism preparedness in rural and urban communities [abstract]. Available at: http://crisp.cit.nih.gov/crisp/crisp_query.generate_screen. Accessed September 14, 2004.

[60] Loeb J. Measurement & bioterrorism preparedness: An impact study [abstract]. Available at: http://crisp.cit.nih.gov/crisp/crisp_query.generate_screen. Accessed September 14, 2004.

[61] Longini I. Containing bioterroist and emerging infectious diseases [abstract]. Available at: http://crisp.cit.nih.gov/crisp/crisp_query.generate_screen. Accessed September 14, 2004.

[62] Hupert N. Modeling US Health Systems' epidemic response capacity [abstract]. Available at: http://crisp.cit.nih.gov/crisp/crisp_query.generate_screen. Accessed September 14, 2004.

[63] Hopkins D. Motherhood, stress, and role strain in junior enlisted women. TriService Nursing Research Program [abstract]. Available at: http://www.usuhs.mil/tsnrp/funded/fy2004/hopkins.html. Accessed September 14, 2004.

[64] Pierce P. Air Force women's health surveillance study [abstract]. Available at: http://www.usuhs.mil/tsnrp/funded/fy1998/piercep.html. Accessed September 14, 2004.

[65] Ross MC. Using after action reports for readiness competency training [abstract]. Available at: http://www.usuhs.mil/tsnrp/funded/fy2003/rossb.html. Accessed September 14, 2004.

[66] Rivers F. Identifying competency skills of PROFIS personnel [abstract]. Available at: http://www.usuhs.mil/tsnrp/funded/fy2002/rivers.html. Accessed September 14, 2004.

[67] McNulty M. Deployed families and their health care needs [abstract]. Available at: http://www.usuhs.mil/tsnrp/funded/fy2000/mcnulty.html. Accessed September 14, 2004.

[68] Williams R. (2004). FICS for sailors: follow-up intervention study [abstract]. Available at: http://www.usuhs.mil/tsnrp/funded/fy2004/williams.html. Accessed September 14, 2004.

Nurs Clin N Am 40 (2005) 565–577

NURSING CLINICS
OF NORTH AMERICA

Hospital Response to Acute-Onset Disasters: The State of the Science in 2005

Mary W. Chaffee, ScD (hon), MS, RN, CNAA, FAAN*

Graduate School of Nursing, Uniformed Services University of the Health Sciences,
Bethesda, MD, USA

ndividuals and communities depend upon hospitals to be able to provide health services in the event of a disaster or other emergency situation. Because of recent terrorist acts in the United States and a steady stream of natural disasters and industrial/transportation disasters, the level of emergency preparedness in US hospitals is a concern. Nurses comprise one of the largest segments of the hospital workforce. Thus, nurses have a significant role to play in hospital disaster response and should be concerned with the development of plans and responses that are rooted in evidence.

WHY EXAMINE THE STATE OF THE SCIENCE?

In simple terms, the state of the science defines what is known about a particular topic at a specific time. For a profession based on science, determining and documenting the state of the science is vital to the growth of knowledge. The current state of the science serves as the platform for generating ideas and research questions that when answered will lead to expanded knowledge in the future (Fig. 1).

The science of hospital emergency preparedness is a body of knowledge in the early stages of development. Indeed, the first US hospitals were not established until the first half of the 19th century and were largely custodial. Nosocomial infection was so rampant that home care was preferred [1]. Since then, urbanization, an explosion in clinical knowledge, and a revolution in technology and computerization have made the contemporary hospital a foundation of emergency preparedness and response.

Professional nursing practice increasingly is evidence-based, as are the practices of medicine, public health, and disaster management. Exploration of knowledge through research continuously expands and changes the body of knowledge incorporated into practice. An examination of the state of the

*8601 Lime Kiln Court, Montgomery Village, MD 20886, USA. *E-mail address:* mwchaffee@aol.com

0029-6465/05/$ – see front matter
doi:10.1016/j.cnur.2005.04.013

Published by Elsevier Inc.
nursing.theclinics.com

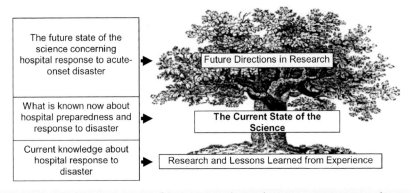

The future state of the science concerning hospital response to acute-onset disaster ▶ Future Directions in Research

What is known now about hospital preparedness and response to disaster ▶ **The Current State of the Science**

Current knowledge about hospital response to disaster ▶ Research and Lessons Learned from Experience

Fig. 1. Model of the current state of the science in hospital response to acute-onset disaster.

science is a vital step on the scientific path. It defines what is known right now. By discovering the gaps in the science and scanning the environment, questions can be asked and answered through research. This ultimately will cause the state of the science, and the practice based on it, to evolve. If one accepts there is much that is unknown, or unproven, about how hospitals respond to disaster, then there is a true need to generate new knowledge.

In the case of the state of the science of how hospitals respond to acute onset disaster, an important assessment was provided by Milsten in his article titled "Hospital responses to acute-onset disasters: a review" published in *Prehospital and Disaster Medicine* in 2000 [2]. Milsten's analysis serves as a stepping-stone, to examine what was known then, to frame an examination of what is known now, and to inspire questions that should be explored to build science in the future.

THE FOUNDATION OF THE CURRENT SCIENCE AS DEFINED BY MILSTEN

Milsten [2] performed a comprehensive review of the literature on how hospitals respond to acute-onset disasters. His review provided an accurate portrayal of what was known at the time about common problems encountered in hospital disaster operations, injury patterns noted in natural disasters, and how that knowledge (lessons learned) can be applied in hospital disaster planning. At the time of the article's development and publication, Milsten was a fellow in emergency medicine at the University of Maryland, Baltimore.

Study selection criteria

Milsten's review of the literature was conducted using the Medline and Healthstar computerized databases. Search terms were not identified. One hundred seven articles published from 1977 through March 1999 were included. Milsten included articles in the review if they "contained information pertaining to a hospital response to a disaster situation or data on specific disaster injury patterns." In Milsten's review of the literature, 69.5% of its content was drawn from the medical literature. Only 5% of the articles were from the nursing literature (Fig. 2).

FINDINGS IN MILSTEN'S STATE OF THE SCIENCE

Milsten identified 107 articles that met his criteria for inclusion in his review, but not all of the articles were research studies or summaries of studies. Some of the articles were case studies presented as 'lessons learned' from an individual's or organization's viewpoint. In addition to the research data and case studies, Milsten presented some content as recommendations for practice that do not appear to be based on evidence. These recommendations usually are stated as "hospitals should. ..." Milsten's analyses can be viewed as a three-legged stool (Fig. 3). His analyses rest on science, lessons learned, and supposition. This perspective may be reflective of the relatively young state of science in hospital emergency preparedness.

Problems identified in Milsten's review

Milsten summarized his findings according to problems that were noted frequently in the literature. Frequently noted problems are highlighted here.

Communications

Milsten described various communications breakdowns documented in hospitals that experienced disasters and referenced several studies done on communications problems in disaster. Failure of telephone-dependent systems was the first problem identified. This is noteworthy, since hospitals remain reliant on telephone systems to communicate internally and externally. Examination of communications problems in hospitals during the past 5 years is important. Communications technology has changed significantly, and the value of multiple back-ups, hand-held radios (walkie-talkies), and wireless Internet should be discerned. Although Milsten described communications problems in disaster, he

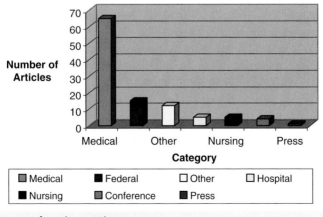

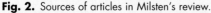

Fig. 2. Sources of articles in Milsten's review.

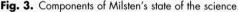

Analysis of the State of the Science
by Milsten (2000)

Evidence from Research

"Lessons Learned" (Case studies)

Recommendations without evidence

Fig. 3. Components of Milsten's state of the science.

did not identify references that address how to mitigate or remedy the situation. He noted Ham radio operators may be a useful resource [2].

Power failures

Milsten [2] identified nine studies or descriptions of hospital power failures and their impact on hospital functions. Hospitals, as energy-intensive businesses, are extremely vulnerable to loss of power. Problems ensuing from power failure include the need to manually ventilate mechanically ventilated patients, problems with elevator transport, and the inability to use infusion pumps, suction machines, and other equipment dependent on a power supply. In addition, the hazard posed to hospital staff by dangling live power lines was mentioned.

In his discussion of power failures, Milsten described many problems related to power failure in hospitals but only once mentioned the concept of back-up power generators. Since 2000, several hospitals have experienced disaster-related partial and total power loss, and these experiences have been published. Greenwald and colleagues [3] and others have documented the impact of the major northeastern US blackout on hospitals.

Water system failures

Hospitals depend upon water systems to provide patient care services. Access to potable water and functional systems to remove waster water are necessary. Disasters can disrupt hospital water systems through physical damage or contamination of water itself. Milsten described various documented hospital disasters where water systems were disrupted. Unlike the section on power failures, he included extensive examples of how hospitals managed the loss of water and mitigated the problem by taking action before a disaster (in the case of hurricanes when early warning was possible).

Hospitals' responses to water loss included closing unused toilet facilities, borrowing water from neighboring, unaffected hospitals, using reverse osmosis water purification units provided by the National Guard, using tanker trucks, pre-arranging vendor deliveries, changing hand washing routines, canceling elective surgeries, and using portable toilet and dialysis machines.

Milsten's review of water system failures is an example of a truly valuable review of the literature. In this section, Milsten described the problems caused by water system failure in hospitals but also detailed actions that damaged hospitals took to deal with the problem of water system loss. These examples are the most valuable part of Milsten's work and can be examined further for application in other hospitals' disaster plans. A description of measures that did not work and why also would have been valuable.

Physical damage to facilities

Milsten provided an analysis of physical damage to hospitals and explained why hospitals are vulnerable to collapse. His review cited several examples of hospital collapses, the consequences, and lessons learned. Additional articles have appeared since Milsten's review that add to this body of knowledge. Several authors, including Parson [4], Nates [5], and Corey [6] described damage and response to flooding from Tropical Storm Allison in 2001. Schultz and colleagues [7] described the damage to a hospital in Los Angeles County from the Northridge earthquake.

Hazardous materials exposure

Milsten discussed the problem of hazardous materials exposures in the United States in general terms. He noted only two examples of hazardous materials exposure impact on hospitals and provided examples of how hospitals can mitigate and manage hazardous materials events. He discussed the sarin terror attack in Tokyo but mentioned the impact on only one hospital. Extensive literature on this attack is available that was not included in Milsten's review.

Hospital evacuation-related problems

Milsten cited 12 articles that described problems related to the physical damage in a hospital and the evacuation process of patients. Significant literature has been published on this area since Milsten's review. Sternberg and colleagues [8] examined all US hospital evacuations during a 28-year period. Meche [9] provided a case study of a hospital's decision to not evacuate during Hurricane Lily. Nates [5] described the failure of all hospital systems, and resulting evacuation of 570 patients, from five hospital buildings following Tropical Storm Allison. Although clinical conditions have obvious differences, there is also value in examining evacuation-related issues of private businesses. Drabek [10] conducted an extensive review of this topic.

Resource allocation and personnel

Milsten included many diverse variables under resource allocation and personnel. His analysis provided a brief review of many issues, including use of volunteers, licensure issues, blood donors, supply problems, and staff absenteeism. Each of these topics is a significant issue and deserves in-depth analysis and study.

Injury patterns

Milsten identified 29 articles that described injury patterns seen in natural disasters, including hurricanes, tornadoes, and earthquakes. Most of these were case studies of an individual facility's experiences. He only identified one article on the impact of bombing. Since Milsten's review, the science has grown in this area. Chou and colleagues [11] and Liang and colleagues [12] studied mortality and morbidity in earthquakes in Asia. Chou analyzed socioeconomic factors and their relation to risk of death, the first exploration of this phenomenon. Because most terror attacks resulting in casualties involve bombing or blast, the study of this phenomenon is vital [13]. Arnold and colleagues [14] compared epidemiologic outcomes of terrorist bombings that produced 30 or more casualties. Thompson and colleagues [15] studied the 574 injuries and 19 deaths in the Khobar Towers bombing. Nufer and Ramirez-Wilson [16] examined clinical complaints of patients after hurricanes Iniki and Andrew.

Hospital disaster plans

Milsten examined the issue of effective disaster planning in hospitals. Again, this topic includes many variables not thoroughly analyzed by Milsten, but an important part of planning. Much knowledge related to exactly what type of planning leads to the most effective outcomes does not exist. Thus one wonders if the recommendations made by Milsten are scientifically based or based on personal opinion.

Hospital disaster plans and lessons learned

The section on hospital disaster plans and lessons learned is perhaps the weakest in Milsten's analysis, for little of it appears rooted in evidence. It did raise an extremely important question: What exactly is a lesson learned? Simon and Teperman [17], Crupi and colleagues [18], Cyganik [19], Langworthy and colleagues [20], and others have published articles that identify lessons learned concerning disaster response. How should researchers approach articles such as these—as factual evidence that expands knowledge—or as stories told from a narrow perspective? A concept analysis of lessons learned is needed.

GAPS IN MILSTEN'S STATE OF THE SCIENCE

Recent research has added much to the knowledge base regarding hospital preparedness and response to disaster. Keim and colleagues [21] studied how well-prepared US hospitals are for chemical terrorism. Milsten and colleagues [22] examined variables affecting medical usage rates in mass gatherings. Greenberg and colleagues [23] studied emergency department preparedness. Treat and colleagues [24] performed an assessment of hospital preparedness for weapons of mass destruction. Keim and Rhyne [25] conducted a pilot study of an emergency preparedness initiative in Oceania. Ciraulo and colleagues [26] surveyed hospital preparedness for terrorism and mass casualty incidents.

Berrios-Torres and colleagues [27] examined disaster worker injury and illness patterns at the World Trade Center. Arnold and colleagues [14] examined clinical outcomes of terrorist bombings.

Hospital preparedness assessment and planning

Milsten presented a section on hospital disaster planning, but he did not note any literature on assessing hospital preparedness, planning strategies, and casualty prediction methods. Articles on these topics have appeared in the literature since Milsten's review. Higgins and colleagues [28] published an article on a hospital assessment tool that was piloted in 116 hospitals. Chaffee and colleagues [29] presented a program designed to assess and strengthen hospital preparedness in US hospitals. Hutchinson, Christopher and colleagues [30] published an article on mass casualty prediction methodology. De Boer [31] examined 416 disasters over a 40-year period using the disaster severity scale. This article was omitted from Milsten's review.

Surge capacity

Milsten's review briefly addressed the concept of surge capacity, the ability of an organization to rapidly increase its operating capability during a disaster. Barbera and colleagues [32] published an article that drew significant attention to weaknesses in US surge capacity. Hick and colleagues [33] published a state of the science review on surge capacity that included strategies for increasing capacity. The Agency for Health care Quality and Research [34] funded a project to examine a model expanding regional surge capacity. Community preparedness, including emergency preparedness funding, was examined by McHugh and colleagues [35]. Developing community surge capacity also was explored by Bekemeier and Dahl [36]. McKenzie and colleagues [37] documented the number and configuration of trauma centers in the United States gaps in coverage. Posner and colleagues [38] presented a strategy to expand burn unit capacity based on work in Israel. The often-overlooked capacity of long-term care facilities was described by Saliba and colleagues [39]. Special problems in surge capacity in rural regions were explored by Gursky [40].

Security

The topic of hospital security was raised by Milsten. Although considered a critical factor in disaster response, little has been published in the 5 years since Milsten's review. Luizzo and Scaglione [41] published an assessment of changes in hospital security since Sept. 11, 2001.

Disaster mental health

Milsten cited one reference in his very brief discussion of mental health needs in disasters. Much literature has been published since Milsten's review, and a debate has occurred concerning the value of critical incident stress management (CISM). Reeves [42] described mental health interventions aboard USNS COMFORT while it was deployed to New York City following the terrorist attacks of Sept. 11, 2001. Stein and colleagues [43] conducted reviewed emotional and behavioral consequences of bioterrorism. Siegel and colleagues [44] demanded new data to accurately estimate mental health capacity requirements in disaster. Mitchell [45] described essential factors in effective psychological response to disaster. Koote [46] examined psychological response to the attacks on the USS STARK and the USS COLE.

Exercises

Milsten's only reference to the importance of exercising hospital disaster plans concerns the need to execute unannounced drills during odd hours and shift changes. Milsten's reference for this statement came from an article on the development of peptic ulcers following an earthquake. Exercising hospital disaster plans is an expensive activity in terms of staff time and preparation and loss of time from delivery of services. Data are needed to determine if indeed hospital personnel who drill perform more effectively during disaster. At least one recent case study supported this assumption. Dacy [47] described his experience as an emergency medicine physician in an emergency department that received 200 injured and burned patients from the Station Nightclub fire in February 2003. Dacy [47] wrote that the hospital mounted a successful disaster response, because it had drilled the units involved in response. Additionally, the disaster occurred at change of shift, and two shifts of nursing personnel were at the facility. This topic has been addressed in the literature though lessons learned articles. Sweeney and colleagues [48] described a regional disaster drill in May 2003 to test multiple facilities in Philadelphia.

Ethics

Larkin and Arnold [49] identified ethical considerations in emergency planning as an important issue. The ethics of evacuation were introduced in a study on evacuation decisions made in hospitals damaged by the California Northridge earthquake. Most facilities evacuated the most seriously ill first; one facility evacuated the most well first because of what they perceived as imminent danger of hospital collapse [7].

Organizational leadership in a crisis

The role of leadership during a disaster recently has gained attention. McCaughrin and Mattammal [50] published an extensive examination of patient care management in a natural disaster. Parsons [51] described components of executive crisis communication skills. Watkins and Bazerman [52] provided perspectives on leadership anticipation of disaster. McKinney and Davis [53] examined the role of human factors on crisis decision performance. Sternberg [54] provided an overview of key concepts in managing uncertainty.

Fatality management

Milsten did not address the need for hospitals to have fatality management plans. This need has emerged as an under-recognized problem in hospital disaster planning. Most US hospitals have extremely limited morgue capacity.

Few have plans to expand morgue capacity through strategies like leasing refrigerated trucks or using ice rinks, and plans to deal with contaminated remains are nearly nonexistent. Nolte and colleagues [55] published an examination of fatality management issues. More study is required in this area.

Health care provider competence

A body of literature is emerging concerning how well prepared US health care providers are to function effectively in disasters. Various factors are being examined in this area, and much in this area requires additional study. Wisniewski and colleagues [56] examined nurses' educational needs. Thorne and colleagues [57] described the need to tailor training to nonclinical hospital workers. Levi and Bregman [58] examined the use of simulation and management games to prepare health system personnel to function effectively in disaster.

Nursing literature

The literature about nursing's role in disaster is expanding. French and colleagues [59] conducted a study of nurses' experiences in hospital disaster response during a Florida hurricane. Suserud and Haljamae [60] conducted a qualitative study of nurses' experiences at disasters sites. Mitani and colleagues [61] examined factors that affect nurse participation in disaster response after an earthquake.

Behavior of the public in disaster

Several articles have appeared since Milsten's review concerning how people behave in a disaster. The concept of convergence (the movement of people toward a disaster site) was explored by Auf der Heide [62] and Cone and colleagues [63]. Glass provided an overview of public behavior in disaster, including the lack of panic generally noted [64].

Other issues also deserve examination to ensure that the highest quality patient care is provided in resource-constrained environments. These issues include the ability of health care providers to protect themselves from threats, triage methods, hospital management of crime scenes and evidence, planned innovation, risk communications, the use of technology in disaster response, disaster care for special populations (eg, pediatrics, geriatrics, or maternity), and incident command. The process of hospital recovery from disasters also requires examination.

VALUE OF THIS REVIEW IN PATIENT CARE

Milsten [2] laid critical groundwork in his 2000 review of the state of the science of hospital disaster response. The review provides an excellent starting point from which to develop further knowledge about the state of the science. Because disaster is such an inherently complex phenomenon, it presents special challenges. Recognizing the need to develop a standardized methodology to approach medical disaster research, the Utstein style has been adapted to medical disaster research [65] (MW Chaffee, unpublished data, 2004).

Several sophisticated statistical analyses have been published by authors in Israel on mass casualty management after terrorist attack. Frykberg [13] provided insightful commentary on these.

> "The validity of the sophisticated statistical analyses. . .is somewhat suspect with regard to our ability to derive any clinically meaningful conclusions from them, in view of the many uncontrollable variables involved in making all the complex decisions being measured. Nonetheless, their attempt to apply science to derive orderly patterns from the apparent chaos and unpredictability of mass casualty events is commendable, and a model we should all follow."

Frykberg's comments are indeed valuable in any state of the science concerning disasters. The number and variety of variables make disaster research challenging but not impossible.

The state of the science concerning how hospitals respond to acute-onset disasters has great significance:

- For patients who may need care when they are most vulnerable
- For health care providers who will be called upon to provide care in complex, uncertain environments
- For health care leaders who will have to make decisions under pressure
- For emergency management planners who work to achieve optimal preparedness with minimum resources
- For legislators who must identify public policy solutions.

Hospitals are the foundation of the US health system and are a critical part of the public health safety net. Although emergency preparedness is an important aspect of hospital operations, it must compete with other priorities. Thus, evidence of what really makes a difference in hospital preparedness is essential. An ongoing examination of the state of the science is essential in building plans and systems based on knowledge.

References

[1] Hollingsworth JR, Hollingsworth EJ. Controversy about American hospitals: funding, ownership, and performance. In: Rothstein WG, editor. Readings in American health care—current issues in socio–historical perspective. Madison (WI): The University of Wisconsin Press; 1995. p. 239–53.

[2] Milsten A. Hospital responses to acute-onset disasters: a review. Prehospital Disaster Med 2000;15(1):32–45.

[3] Greenwald PW, Rutherford AF, Green RA, et al. Emergency department visits for home medical device failure during the 2003 North America blackout. Acad Emerg Med 2004;11(7):786–9.

[4] Parson E. (2002). 1000 year flood paralyzes Texas Medical Center. Available at: www.ecmweb.com/microsites/magazinearticle.asp. Accessed September 10, 2004.

[5] Nates JL. Combined external and internal hospital disaster: Impact and response in a Houston trauma center intensive care unit. Crit Care Med 2004;32(3):686–90.

[6] Corey F. What we learned when Allison turned out the big light. Crit Care Med 2004;32(3):884–5.

[7] Schultz CH, Koenig KL, Lewis RJ. Implications of hospital evacuation after the Northridge, California, earthquake. N Engl J Med 2003;348(14):1349–55.

[8] Sternberg E, Lee GC, Huard D. Counting crises: US hospital evacuations, 1971–1999. Prehospital Disaster Med 2004;19(2):150–7.

[9] Meche VC. Lafayette (Louisiana) General Medical Center responds to Hurricane Lily by riding the storm out. J Emerg Nurs 2003;29(6):551–4.

[10] Drabek TE. Disaster warning and evacuation responses by private business employees. Disasters 2001;25(1):76–95.

[11] Chou Y, Huang N, Lee C, et al. Who is at risk of death in an earthquake? Am J Epidemiol 2004;160(7):688–95.

[12] Liang N, Shih Y, Shih F, et al. Disaster epidemiology and medical response in the Chi-Chi earthquake in Taiwan. Ann Emerg Med 2001;38(11):549–55.

[13] Frykberg ER. Principles of mass casualty management following terrorist disasters. [editorial]. Ann Surg 2003;239(3):319–21.

[14] Arnold JL, Halpern P, Tsai MC, et al. Mass casualty terrorist bombings: a comparison of outcomes by bombing type. Ann Emerg Med 2004;43(2):263–73.

[15] Thompson D, Brown S, Mallonnee S, et al. Fatal and nonfatal injuries among US Air Force personnel resulting from the terrorist bombing of the Khobar Towers. The Journal of Trauma, Injury. Infection and Critical Care 2004;57(2):208–15.

[16] Nufer KE, Ramirez-Wilson G. A comparison of patient needs following two hurricanes. Prehospital Disaster Med 2004;19(1):146–9.

[17] Simon R, Teperman S. The World Trade Center attack: lessons for disaster management. Crit Care 2001;5(6):318–20.

[18] Crupi RS, Asnis DS, Lee CC, et al. Meeting the challenge of bioterrorism: lessons learned from West Nile virus and anthrax. Am J Emerg Med 2003;21(1):77–9.

[19] Cyganik KA. Disaster preparedness in Virginia Hospital Center–Arlington after September 11, 2001. Disaster Manag Response 2003;1(3):80–6.

[20] Langworthy MJ, Sabra J, Gould M. Terrorism and blast phenomena: lessons learned from the attack on the USS Cole (DDG67). Clin Orthop 2004;42(2):82–7.

[21] Keim ME, Pesik N, Twum-Danso NA. Lack of hospital preparedness for chemical terrorism in a major US city: 1996–2000. Prehospital Disaster Med 2003;18(3):193–9.

[22] Milsten AM, Seaman KG, Liu P, et al. Variables influencing medical usage rates, injury patterns and levels of care for mass gatherings. Prehospital Disaster Med 2003;18(4):334–45.

[23] Greenberg MI, Jurgens SM, Gracely EJ. Emergency department preparedness for the evaluation and treatment of victims of biological or chemical terrorist attack. J Emerg Med 2002;22(3):273–8.

[24] Treat KN, Williams JM, Furbee PM, et al. Hospital preparedness for weapons of mass destruction incidents: an initial assessment. Ann Emerg Med 2001;38(5):562–5.

[25] Keim ME, Rhyne GJ. The CDC Pacific emergency health initiative: a pilot study of emergency preparedness in Oceania. Emerg Med 2001;13:157–64.

[26] Ciraulo DL, Frykberg ER, Feliciano DV, et al. A survey assessment of the level of preparedness for domestic terrorism and mass casualty incidents among Eastern Association for the Surgery of Trauma members. J Trauma 2004;56(5):1033–41.

[27] Berrios-Torres SI, Greenko JA, Phillips M, et al. World Trade Center rescue worker injury and illness surveillance, New York, 2001. Am J Prev Med 2003;25(2):79–87.

[28] Higgins W, Wainright C, Lu N, et al. Assessing hospital preparedness using an instrument based on the mass casualty disaster plan checklist: results of a statewide survey. Am J Infect Control 2004;32(6):327–32.

[29] Chaffee MW, Miranda SM, Padula RM, et al. DVATEX: Navy medicine's innovative approach to improving hospital emergency preparedness. Journal of Emergency Preparedness 2004;2(1):26–32.

[30] Hutchinson R, Christopher G, Mughal MA, et al. Mass casualty prediction: by the numbers. Available at: www.mmt-kmi.com/archive_article.cfm?DocID=59. Accessed September 3, 2004.

[31] De Boer J. Tools for evaluating disasters: preliminary results of some hundreds of disasters. Eur J Emerg Med 1997;4:107–10.

[32] Barbera JA, Mcintyre AG, DeAtley CA. (2002). Ambulances to nowhere: America's short-fall in medical preparedness for catastrophic terrorism. Available at: www.homelandsecurity.org/journal/displayarticle.asp?article=46. Accessed October 20, 2004.

[33] Hick JL, Hanfling D, Burstein JL, et al. Health care facility and community strategies for patient care surge capacity. Ann Emerg Med 2004;44:253–61.

[34] Agency for Healthcare Research and Quality. Rocky Mountain regional care model for bioterrorist events. Available at: www.ahrq.gov/research/altsites.htm. Accessed October 20, 2004.

[35] McHugh M, Stalti AB, Felland LE. How prepared are Americans for public health emergencies? Twelve communities weigh in. Health Aff 2004;23(3):201–9.

[36] Bekemeier B, Dahl J. Turning point sets the stage for emergency preparedness planning. J Public Health Manag Pract 2003;9(5):377–83.

[37] McKenzie EJ, Hoyt DB, Sacra JC, et al. National inventory of hospital trauma centers. JAMA 2003;289(12):1515–22.

[38] Posner Z, Admi H, Menashe N. Ten-fold expansion of a burn unit in mass casualty: how to recruit the nursing staff. Disaster Manage Response 2003;1(4):100–4.

[39] Saliba D, Buchanan J, Kington RS. Function and response of nursing facilities during community disaster. Am J Public Health 2004;94(8):1436–41.

[40] Gursky EA. Hometown hospitals—the weakest link? Report commissioned by the National Defense University Center for Technology and National Security Policy. Arlington (VA): Anser Institute 2004.

[41] Luizzo AJ, Scaglione B. How has hospital security changed since 9/11? J Healthc Prot Manage 2004;20(2):44–8.

[42] Reeves JJ. Perspectives on disaster mental health intervention from the USNS Comfort. Mil Med 2002;167(Suppl 9):90–2.

[43] Stein BD, Tanielian TL, Eisenman DP, et al. Emotional and behavioral consequences of bioterrorism: planning a public health response. Milbank Q 2004;82(3):413–55.

[44] Siegel CE, Laska E, Meisner M. Estimating capacity requirements for mental health services after a disaster has occurred: a call for new data. Am J Public Health 2004;94(4):582–5.

[45] Mitchell JT. Essential factors for effective psychological response to disasters and others crises. Int J Emerg Ment Health 1999;1(1):51–8.

[46] Koote AF. Psychosocial response to disaster: the attacks on the Stark and the Cole. Med Confl Surviv 2002;18(1):44–58.

[47] Dacy MJ. The Rhode Island nightclub fire. Presented at the meeting of the National Disaster Medical System. Dallas (TX), April 19, 2004.

[48] Sweeney B, Jasper E, Gates E. Large-scale urban disaster drill involving an explosion: lessons learned by an academic medical center. Disaster Manag Response 2004;2(3):87–90.

[49] Larkin GL, Arnold J. Ethical considerations in emergency planning, preparedness, and response to acts of terrorism. Prehospital Disaster Med 2003;18(3):170–8.

[50] McCaughrin WC, Mattammal M. Perfect storm: organizational management of patient care under natural disaster conditions. Journal of Heathcare Management 2003; 48(5):295–308.

[51] Parsons PJ. Communicating strategically in a crisis. Healthc Exec 2002;17(6):56–7.

[52] Watkins MD, Bazerman MH. Predictable surprises: the disasters you should have seen coming. Harvard Business Review 2003;81(3):72–80.

[53] McKinney EH, Davis KJ. Effects of deliberate practice on crisis decision performance. Hum Factors 2003;45(3):436–45.

[54] Sternberg E. Planning for resilience in hospital internal disaster. Prehospital Disaster Med 2003;18(4):291–300.

[55] Nolte KB, Hanzlick RL, Payne DC, et al. Medical examiners, coroners and biologic terrorism. MMWR Morb Mortal Wkly Rep 2004;53(RR08):1–27.

[56] Wisniewski R, Dennik-Champion G, Peltier JW. Emergency preparedness competencies—assessing nurses' educational needs. J Nurs Adm 2004;34(10):475–80.

[57] Thorne CD, Oliver M, Al-Ibrahim M, et al. Terrorism- preparedness training for nonclinical hospital workers. J Occup Environ Med 2004;46(7):668–76.

[58] Levi L, Bregman D. Simulation and management games for training command and control in emergencies. Stud Health Technol Inform 2003;95:783–7.

[59] French ED, Sole ML, Byers JF. A comparison of nurses' needs/concerns and hospital disaster plans following Florida's Hurricane Floyd. J Emerg Nurs 2002;28(2):111–7.

[60] Suserud B, Haljamae H. Acting at a disaster site: experiences expressed by Swedish nurses. J Adv Nurs 1997;25:155–62.

[61] Mitani S, Kuboyama K, Shirakawa T. Nursing in sudden-onset disasters: factors and information that affect participation. Prehospital Disaster Med 2003;18(4):359–66.

[62] Auf der Heide E. Convergence behavior in disasters. Ann Emerg Med 2003;41(4):463–6.

[63] Cone DC, Weit SD, Bogucki S. Convergent volunteerism. Ann Emerg Med 2003; 41(4):457–62.

[64] Glass TA. (2003). Understanding public response to disasters. Public Health Rep 2003;116(Suppl 2):69–73.

[65] Sundnes KO, Birnbaum ML. (2003). Conceptual framework of disasters. Prehospital Disaster Med 2003;17(Suppl 3):1–14.

Nurs Clin N Am 40 (2005) 579–586

NURSING CLINICS
OF NORTH AMERICA

The Human Factors in a Disaster

Kevin Davies, RRC, MA, RN, PGCE*,
Ray Higginson, BN, RN, PGCE

School of Care Sciences, University of Glamorgan, Glyntaff, Pontypridd, South Wales,
UK CF37 1DL

"The term 'natural disasters' has become an increasingly anachronistic misnomer. In reality, it is human behaviour that transforms natural hazards into what should be called unnatural disasters." (Kofi Annan, 1999).

For as long as people have inhabited the earth's surface, they have been subject to the forces of nature. With time, people have learned how to adapt to the environment and to reduce risks associated with earthquakes, temperature extremes, storms, and fires. People have learned how to read the skies, weather, and seas and to use precautionary survival skills and to avoid further victimization.

The relationship between people and the earth has been a dynamic process. In a study of 38 recorded disaster events that occurred in the twentieth century, researchers found that 17,985,018 lives were lost in relation to the disasters [1]. Over the latter part of the century, the World Disasters Report, 2002 [2] noted a change in the trend. "In the 1970s, natural disasters alone claimed nearly 2 million lives; by the 1990s this had fallen to under 800,000. But this is still a terrible and premature loss of life. Meanwhile, those affected—whether left injured, homeless or hungry—tripled to 2 billion during the past decade" (p. 1).

Planners are continually looking for means to decrease the morbidity and mortality of disasters. In retrospect, many events could have been predicted by measuring rainfall, monitoring environmental changes, or instigating more sophisticated atmospheric monitoring systems. Yet one theme of disasters should receive greater attention. It is not coincidental that most disaster victims are from poor, third-world areas [3]. This article highlights the relationship of human factors that can be found with third-world disasters and reviews interventions that have been used to reduce illness, injuries and deaths.

Disasters are made worse when the forces of nature exceed a person's ability to avoid or survive those forces. It stands to reason that any additional factors that influence a person's ability to handle stressors will contribute to a greater loss of health or life. Additional factors include poor nutrition, contaminated

*Corresponding author. E-mail address: kdavies@glam.ac.uk (K. Davies).

0029-6465/05/$ – see front matter   © 2005 Elsevier Inc. All rights reserved.
doi:10.1016/j.cnur.2005.04.004   nursing.theclinics.com

water, and a lack of basic health care or community infrastructure to help funnel aid. Kofi Annan was calling attention to the hidden human factors that work to further victimize people, such as inhabiting unsafe buildings, concentrating populations on unstable ground or near flood plains, and stripping natural protection by overusing land. Still other behaviors (eg, civil war or ethic conflicts) strip people of their ability to raise animals, farm the land, educate the masses, or maintain intact family units.

Third-world disasters also can be influenced by the developed world. The twenty-first century trend toward globalization of manufacturing does not offer the same financial security for all countries. This model consists of developed nations exporting manufacturing to the third world to lower production costs. Savings and profits are achieved by exploiting workers with low wages and poor housing. Large profits make the developed nations depend more on third-world imports [4]. Overall, workers experience further poverty, become resentful, and contribute to the destabilization of their governments. The environmental changes associated with globalization also are suspected of contributing to health care threats and contributing to climate changes [5].

HOW PEOPLE CONTRIBUTE TO DISASTERS

A review of previous disasters demonstrates that many natural events could have been predicted by measuring rainfall and environmental climate changes. In third-world disasters, additional man-made factors such as wars, inequalities in wealth distribution, inadequately structured social welfare programs, and poverty are not identified immediately, yet could contribute to an increased human toll. Misdistribution of wealth, the rise of the corporation, the third-world debt crisis, militarization, and wars have contributed to increases in poverty, overcrowding, famine, and weather extremes [6]. Several common themes have been found and are summarized in Box 1.

Failure to provide social, economic, and health infrastructure

Fara [7] investigated the claim that natural disasters are seldom totally natural. Namibia is a country with high temperatures, harsh environment, and farming conditions that make it vulnerable to frequent droughts. Clearly, better planning would not stimulate rainfall. When examining the vulnerability of Namibians, however, it was discovered that poverty was important in how people experience and deal with the problems of drought. The indigenous people live in poverty because of discriminatory land and labor policies, an extractive economy, and restrictive trade practices. If they are to successfully coexist with the challenges of their environment, they need sound economic and social planning [7,8].

Classification of victims

Civil and cross-border conflicts have exacerbated the effects of drought, including the urgent need to distribute food and humanitarian aid. Every year, hundreds of thousands of people flee their homes because of war and conflict

Box 1: Examples of human behaviors that affect morbidity and mortality associated with natural disasters

Behaviors that increase human loss
Failure to provide social, economic and health infrastructure
Classification of victims as refugees versus internally displaced persons
Exposure to environmental hazards

International attempts to diminish human loss
Humanitarian aid agencies work directly with victims of disasters.
• International governmental organizations (IGOs)
• Nongovernmental organizations (NGOs)
International collaboration efforts
• Medecins Sans Frontieres annual list of disaster-prone areas
• Red Cross and Red Crescent working with other NGOs to develop the Sphere Project, to create a humanitarian charter and minimum standards for disaster care
International laws
• The International Federation of the Red Cross (IFRC) raises debate and discussion regarding development of international humanitarian law.
• The United Nations has created the template, Millennium Development Goals, to help all nations to raise the quality of life.

[9], and their status as a refugee or internally displaced person is important. Refugees have formal recognition with the United Nations (UN). The UN is legally obligated under international law for the welfare of refugees. Internally displaced persons have no such recognition and often find themselves at the mercy and whim of various warlords.

Ethiopia experienced a drought, failed crops, and famine during a time when the country was engaged in a boarder war with Eritrea. The country dedicated resources to fight the war, which took away from efforts to build an infrastructure to collect and save sufficient water during good rainy seasons. The Ethiopian government knows when the light and heavy rains are expected each year; light rains appear in February, followed by heavier rains in June [10]. If these rains fail, then crops are depleted, and famine ensues. Knowing that a poor February rainfall is indicative of low June rainfalls should allow disaster relief agencies to act and prepare for any consequent drought. Without the proper infrastructure, however, water cannot be saved, and predictions cannot be acted upon effectively. The World Health Organization (WHO) estimated that 15 million Ethiopians would die between 2003 and 2004 from a malaria epidemic, because the country was unable to care for, treat, or store in a proper manner what little water it did have [10].

Exposure to environmental hazards

The compounding effects of an inadequate infrastructure are demonstrated further in the Sudan. After months of endless sun, Sudan famine victims have to contend with periodic rains and flash floods. Sun-baked soil does not soak up rainfall; flash floods occur, swamp airstrips, and jeopardize food and aid camps [11]. No matter how well-prepared aid agencies are, without properly constructed and well-maintained roads and airstrips, they will not be able to reach certain destinations.

Bangladesh is a poor and disaster-prone country that experiences regular cyclones and flooding from monsoon rains that occur every year in June. In 2003, many houses were flooded, causing deaths among young children and vulnerable adults [12]. The flooding covered about 25,000 acres of rice plantations and was aggravated by India releasing tons of water from the Farakka Dam north of Chapai Nawabganj during the monsoon.

APPROACHES USED TO REDUCE WORLDWIDE DISASTERS

International humanitarian aid agencies

Historically, people have responded to disasters by forming an organization that addresses the postevent needs of the victims (Table 1). Paradoxically, it seems that wars have had a direct influence on producing disasters and also stimulating interventions to overcome the consequences. In 1859, Henri Dunant, a Swiss national, reported witnessing the slaughter in the Battle of Solforino [13]. Later, Dunant published "A Memory of Solferino," which paved the way for the eventual formation of the International Committee of the Red Cross (ICRC) in 1880 [14]. During the twentieth century, there were two world wars and several smaller conflicts and civil wars. Concurrently, there

Table 1
Distinguishing between nongovernmental organizations, intergovernmental organizations, and nongovernmental humanitarian agencies

Nongovernmental organization	Intergovernmental organization	Nongovernmental humanitarian agencies
Organizations that may be national or international but are separate and independent of their country's government	Organizations that are constituted by more than one government	Independent organizations, specifically those involved in disaster response
Examples	Examples	Examples
MSF	UN	ICRC
Concern	WHO	IFRC and RCS
Worldvision	OECD	National Red Cross and Red Crescent Societies
Tearfund	USAID	
Oxfam		
Merlin		

was also a dramatic rise in the number of IGOs and NGOs. In 1909, there 37 IGOs and 167 NGOs; by 1997, there were 260 IGOs and 5472 NGOs [1].

The growth and expansion of IGOs and NGOs is related to several factors. Among those is a sense of protection that people feel from the protocols and conventions that guide their interventions. The organizations are allowed to operate within defined limits and tend to be accepted by all sides. Unfortunately, the increasingly large number of organizations attempting to address worldwide disasters has led to a lack of coordination, duplication of effort, and a waste of resources. Indeed, many organizations still eschew any collaborating effort, claiming that to collaborate will hinder their nonpartisan stance or ethos.

One method to prepare for disasters is to be aware of areas that are at high risk. Many international humanitarian aid agencies share what they have learned to help the rest of the world to focus prevention efforts. Medecins Sans Frontieres (MSF) [15], also referred to as Doctors Without Borders, issues an annual list of under-reported new humanitarian stories of the year. MSF has identified Burundi, Chechnya, China, and Colombia as new disaster-prone areas. MSF's work serves to alert the world about disadvantaged people when the public press fails to provide sufficient coverage to raise concern. The catastrophic man-made famine that claimed thousands of lives in oil-rich Angola and the war in Liberia received little or no television coverage. In most instances, the coverage does not include issues of displacement, disease, and starvation in highly vulnerable groups.

International collaboration

The Sphere Project [16] was launched in 1997 and is the result of the Red Cross and Red Crescent movement and several NGOs. Their work has developed in phases. During the first phase (1997 to 1998), a preliminary edition of a Sphere handbook was developed, including the Humanitarian Charter and Minimum Standards for the care sectors of water supply and sanitation, nutrition, food aid, shelter and site management, and health services. The minimum standards are "...an attempt to describe the level of disaster assistance to which all people have a right—regardless of political, ethnic or geographical specificity." During the second phase (1998 to 2000), planners focused on activities that would translate a commitment to quality and accountability in humanitarian practice into a reality. During the third phase (2000 to 2004), the project revised the handbook, conducted evaluations of their efforts, and conducted pilot projects.

The Sphere project addresses the concern that not all organizations can meet the minimum standards. "...Some indicators may not be attainable by your organization in a given context. This does not necessarily mean that the organization is inefficient or irresponsible..." Other authors have argued that standards of this kind are based on notions of human rights and are something to aspire to. Crucially stipulating principles of practice and participation may have implications for those delivering aid [17,18].

International laws

The IFRC [18] has attempted to engender debate and discussion regarding development of international humanitarian law. The laws would apply to disasters that are not a result of warfare. The IFRC sees the Sphere Project as a "body of . . .international law in the making." It has not been determined how any type of international law could be enforced [17]. The debate continues with reports and discussion on humanitarian action for which accounts can be made [19,20]. Whereas embracing a legal structure may be attractive in the West, it inevitably will fall foul of many ethnic, religious, tribal, and constitutional objections.

In September 2000, the United Nations organized a meeting with the leaders of 189 countries to identify millennium development goals for the year 2015. The UN's goals are intended to reduce poverty, hunger, maternal and child deaths, and spread of HIV and AIDS; and advance primary education and gender equality and promote environmentally sustainable development [21]. The United Nations has helped countries to change their internal laws by integrating the Millennium development goals into their national development frameworks. Over 70 countries have adopted poverty reduction as their main strategic goal. The UN secretary general issues an annual report on the progress of the goals, and a comprehensive review is planned for this year. As an example of the work that has been done under the goals, a program in Nairobi has helped other African countries to undertake forestation projects and offer education on environmentally friendly and sustainable land-use.

Clearly, the list of potentially destructive human behaviors must be considered when planners attempt to identify factors that contribute to the destructiveness of a disaster. Other hidden factors include population and re-productive health issues, the rights of women and children, and the need for improved education for those most vulnerable. In an almost Maslow-type hierarchy, sustainable development cannot be achieved until other basic issues are addressed.

If poverty is to be eased, economic issues will have to be addressed, and there are opportunities to reduce Africa's domestic marketing costs [10]. Port fees can be reduced; transport costs through ports can be reduced, and the timing of fertilizer clearance from a port can be coordinated with up-country transport. Inland transport of goods can be expedited with better rails and roads and reduced fuel taxes. Traders could reduce costs if government input distribution programs were more certain.

SUMMARY

Third-world disasters tend to have common features that involve the victims (eg, impoverished, uneducated, and exploited), countries (eg, lack commercial and public health infrastructure, civil war, and ethnic fighting), and multiple international interventions (eg, classification of victims; assistance from of IGOs and NGOs; world leaders setting global standards; and encouraging efforts to stem root causes of poverty, disease, and famine). International health care professionals can work with specialists in other fields to identify and predict potential areas of real need. The Sphere Project addresses standards; however, the standards are not legally binding on nations. The United Nations has encouraged nations to consider socioeconomic issues, such as globalization of world markets, huge national debt, and the status of refugees and internally displaced persons.

Disasters are complex, multi-faceted phenomena and are more than simply a flood or a famine. Although debate continues on root causes, disaster relief practitioners can help focus attention on the disproportionate humanitarian suffering experienced by vulnerable third-world populations. Just as world markets are globalizing their operations, so should health care providers. Future disaster care goals should include: preventing victimization, developing rapid assistance to victims, and greater coordination of international efforts to plan and implement, appropriately target, and ethically deliver a high standard of culturally appropriate health care.

References

[1] Ryan J, Mahoney PF, Greaves I, et al. Catastrophes—natural and man-made disasters. In: Ryan J, Mahoney PF, Greaves I, et al, editors. Conflict and catastrophe medicine. London: Springer; 2000. p. 27–48.

[2] World Health Organization. Conflicts and disasters: a world health report. Geneva (Switzerland): World Health Organization; 2002.

[3] World Health Organization. Refugee and internationally displaced populations. Flows, occasions and priorities for assistance. Geneva (Switzerland): World Health Organization; 2002.

[4] International Federation of the Red Cross. World disasters report. International Federation of Red Cross and Red Crescent Societies. Geneva (Switzerland): International Federation of the Red Cross; 1998.

[5] Goldin I, Knudsen O, van der Mensbrugghe D. Trade liberalisation: global economic implications. Paris: Organisation for Economic Cooperation and Development; 1990.

[6] Economist. A great yarn.thread of life, death of money. Available at: www.economist.com/display.cfm-id/yarn. Accessed February 9, 2004.

[7] Fara K. How natural are natural disasters? Vulnerability to drought in southern areas. Disaster 2000;15(3):209–26.

[8] Ryan JM, Lumley JSP. And finally....failed states and failing states. Trauma 2000;2(3): 231–5.

[9] Bhatt M. Mapping vulnerability, participatory tool kits. In: Ingleton J, editor. Natural disasters management. London: Tudor Rose; 1999.

[10] Jayne TS, Govereh J, Wanzala M, Demeke M. Fertilizer market development. A comparative analysis between Ethiopia, Kenya and Zambia. Food Policy 2003;28(4): 293–316.

[11] Brill J. Needed rain comes fast and furious in volunteer states. Disaster relief.org 1998.

[12] World Health Organization. $341 million needed for the health 45 million people in the developed world. Geneva (Switzerland): World Health Organization; 2003.

[13] Wylly HC. The campaign of Magenta and Solferino 1859. London: Spellmount Publishers; 1997.

[14] Henry DJ. A memory of Solferino. London: Cassell; 1947.

[15] MSF. The top ten underreported disasters of 2002. Available at: www.msf.org/countries/page.cfm. Accessed February 9, 2004.

[16] The Sphere Project. Humanitarian charter and minimum standards in disaster response. Available at: http://www.sphereproject.org/handbook/index.htm. Accessed February 9, 2004.

[17] Slim H. Future imperatives? Quality, standards and human rights. Report of a study to explore quality standards for the British Overseas aid group (BOAG). Centre for Development and Emergency Practice (CENDEP). Oxford (United Kingdom): Oxford Brookes University; 1998.

[18] International Federation of the Red Cross. World Disaster Report. International Federation of Red Cross and Red Crescent Societies. Geneva. 2000. 145–157.

[19] Perrin P. War and accountability—a framework. Forum. Geneva (Switzerland): International Federation of the Red Cross; 2002.

[20] Van Brabant K. Accountable humanitarian action: an overview of recent trends. Forum. 2002. Geneva (Switzerland): ICRC; 2002.

[21] Attawel K. Strike out for the millennium goals. The health exchange. Available at: http://www.un.org/millenniumgoals. Accessed February 9, 2004.

Nurs Clin N Am 40 (2005) 587–593

NURSING CLINICS
OF NORTH AMERICA

INDEX

Note: Page numbers of article titles are in **boldface** type.

0029-6465/05/$ – see front matter
doi:10.1016/S0029-6465(05)00068-X

Changing Your Address?

Make sure your subscription changes too! When you notify us of your new address, you can help make our job easier by including an exact copy of your Clinics label number with your old address (see illustration below.) This number identifies you to our computer system and will speed the processing of your address change. Please be sure this label number accompanies your old address and your corrected address—you can send an old Clinics label with your number on it or just copy it exactly and send it to the address listed below.

We appreciate your help in our attempt to give you continuous coverage. Thank you.

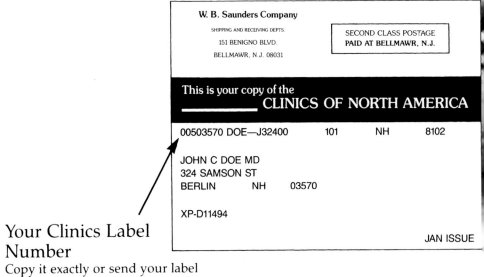

W. B. Saunders Company

SHIPPING AND RECEIVING DEPTS.
151 BENIGNO BLVD.
BELLMAWR, N.J. 08031

SECOND CLASS POSTAGE
PAID AT BELLMAWR, N.J.

This is your copy of the
_____ CLINICS OF NORTH AMERICA

| 00503570 DOE—J32400 | 101 | NH | 8102 |

JOHN C DOE MD
324 SAMSON ST
BERLIN   NH   03570

XP-D11494

JAN ISSUE

Your Clinics Label Number
Copy it exactly or send your label along with your address to:
W.B. Saunders Company, Customer Service
Orlando, FL 32887-4800
Call Toll Free 1-800-654-2452

Please allow four to six weeks for delivery of new subscriptions and for processing address changes.